Foundations in SPORTS THERAPY

Dale Forsdyke

Adam Gledhill

Nikki Mackay

Kate Randerson

www.pearsonschoolsandfe.co.uk

✓ Free online support
✓ Useful weblinks
✓ 24 hour online ordering

0845 630 44 44

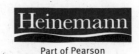

Heinemann

Part of Pearson

Heinemann is an imprint of Pearson Education Limited, Edinburgh Gate, Harlow, Essex, CM20 2JE.

www.pearsonschoolsandfecolleges.co.uk

Heinemann is a registered trademark of Pearson Education Limited

Text © Pearson Education Limited 2011

Designed by Brian Melville

Typeset by Brian Melville

Original illustrations © Pearson Education Limited 2011

Illustrated by Pearson Education, Oxford Designers and Illustrators and Brian Melville

Cover design by Brian Melville

Picture research by Susannah Prescott

Cover photo © Getty Images: Ashley Karyl

The rights of Dale Forsdyke, Adam Gledhill, Nikki Mackay and Kate Randerson to be identified as authors of this work have been asserted by them in accordance with the Copyright, Designs and Patents Act 1988.

First published 2011

14 13 12 11

10 9 8 7 6 5 4 3 2 1

British Library Cataloguing in Publication Data

A catalogue record for this book is available from the British Library

ISBN 978 0 435 04685 9

Printed in Spain by Graficas Estella

Websites

There are links to relevant websites in this book. In order to ensure that the links are up to date and that the links work we have made the links available on our website at www.pearsonhotlinks.co.uk. Search for this title Foundations in Sports Therapy or ISBN 9780435046859.

Contents

Author acknowledgements

Dale Forsdyke

Thank you to my wife Sophie for her constant support through the writing process and in life generally, and also to my daughter Isla who is a welcome distraction and helps puts things into perspective.

Adam Gledhill

Thank you to my family and Amy for all their support and patience throughout my writing of this book, and thank you to my nephew Jack whose smiles and giggles were a very welcome distraction.

Nikki Mackay

Thank you to my fiancé, mum, dad, sister and wonderful nephews. Many thanks also to my friends and mentors Kate Randerson, Julie Hancock and Lynne Evans for their wisdom and advice over the years. Thank you to Northampton Saints, particularly Kiera Ruddy, Nick Johnston and Chris Wearmouth, for their permission and support in writing Chapter 17. And finally thank you to Francesca Heslop, for her expertise as publisher.

Kate Randerson

Thanks to all at Bramley Phoenix RFC: to the Presidents past and present, Lady Chair, Mike Ryan, Jack Robinson, Steve Langton and Stuart MacPherson. Thank you to all the captains and players over the past ten years for including me in the team, for being great competitors and for keeping Rugby Union at a local level an important part of the community. Last but certainly not least, thanks to my husband for his uncomplaining patience and understanding.

Acknowledgements

The author and publisher would like to thank the following individuals and organisations for permission to reproduce, materials and photographs:

Chapter 17: Case study with kind permission of Northampton Saints RFC.

p.81: Body Mass Index nomogram, reprinted by permission from Macmillan Publishers Ltd: *International journal of Obesity*, Bray, G.A. (1978). Definition, measurements and classification of the syndromes of obesity, 2, 99–112, copyright 1978.

p.136: The differences between walking and sprinting, printed with permission from McGraw-Hill Australia: Brukner, P. & Khan, K. (2006). *Clinical Sports Medicine (3rd edition)*, p.48

p.143: Stress injury model of sports injury from Williams, J.M., and Andersen, M.B. (1998). Psychosocial antecedents of sport injury: Review and critique of the stress injury model. *Journal of Applied Sport Psychology*, 10, 5–25, reprinted by permission of Taylor & Francis Group, http://www.informaworld.com.

p.145: Cognitive appraisal model of psychological adjustment to sports injury from Brewer, B.W. (1994). Review and critique of models of psychological adjustment to athletic injury. *Journal of applied sport psychology*, 6, 87–100, reprinted by permission of Taylor & Francis Group, http://www.informaworld.com.

Corbis: Rubberball 1, 21, 36, 50, 62, 77, 93, 105, 120, 131, 141, 156, 166, 176, 187, 193, 199, Sullivan 118; **DJO UK Ltd**: 72; **DK Images**: Ruth Jenkinson 73; **Fotolia.com**: PA 48; **Getty Images**: 34, Bryn Lennon 129, David Rogers 165, Ryan McVay/Digital Vision 48b, Shaun Botterill 200, 201, Thomas Barwick/The Image Bank 91; **iStockphoto**: Philartphace 45, 102, Stockstyle 57; **Marshcouch Treatment Couches**: 171; **Pearson Education Ltd**: Gareth Boden 60, Studio8 42, 58t, 58l, 58r, 59, **Photolibrary.com**: Uppercut Images 167; **Rex Features**: Offside 146; **Shutterstock.com**: Brasiliao 22, Doug James 139, Howard Sandler 19, Paul Hakimata Photography 174, Pete Saloutos 103, Robert Kneschke 126, Tosoth 46, Val Thoermer 153. All other images © Pearson Education Limited. (Key: b-bottom; c-centre; l-left; r-right; t-top)

Every effort has been made to contact copyright holders of material reproduced in this book. We apologise in advance for any unintentional omissions. Any omissions will be rectified in subsequent printings if notice is given to the publishers.

About the authors

Dale Forsdyke has 11 years experience of teaching and managing Higher Education programmes in a Further Education setting. He has helped write BTEC Higher National Diploma programmes and has written a Society of Sports Therapists accredited Foundation Degree in Sports Therapy run at York College. Dale has worked with a number of sports clubs in various capacities and provided sports massage therapy privately and at the London Marathon.

Adam Gledhill has nine years experience teaching sports and exercise sciences and sports therapy courses across Further and Higher Education. He has contributed to the development of a Foundation Degree in Sports Therapy that is currently accredited by the Society of Sports Therapists. Adam has co-authored ten publications within sport or sport and exercise sciences, works as an educational consultant for a national consultancy firm and is currently working towards a PhD in Sport Psychology.

Nikki Mackay has her own Sports Injury Consultancy and Wellbeing clinic working with elite, professional and recreational sports people and clubs. She also works as an educational consultant, freelance lecturer and examiner. Nikki has recently been appointed Chief Verifier for Sport, Active and Leisure, is an assessment associate and writer, and an external examiner for two leading educational awarding bodies. She has lectured across a range of programmes and module subjects, including lecturing on teacher training programmes, mentoring and contributing to staff development programmes. Specialising in Sports Therapy she led the writing and validation of FdSc and BSc Sports Therapy programme by University of Northampton.

Kate Randerson is a Senior Lecturer in Sports and Exercise Therapy at Leeds Metropolitan University. With over 25 years teaching experience she has been involved in the design, delivery and progression of new sports therapy courses in both Further and Higher Education. Her research interests are pitch side and emergency management of the injured athlete, sports massage and rehabilitation. Kate is also the appointed sports therapist for a local amateur Rugby Union Team working with the players and coaches attending matches and training sessions.

Introduction

Who is this book for?

This book is an essential guide for students studying a foundation degree in Sports Therapy and BTEC Higher Nationals in Sport and Sport and Exercise Sciences.

About foundation degrees

Your foundation degree should enable you to develop the intermediate higher education skills that characterise high-quality graduates needed in the labour market and should integrate academic and work-based learning. It is likely that your foundation degree will have been developed in collaboration with employers and have a focus on the development of work-related skills and knowledge and their direct application to the workplace.

As a foundation degree graduate you should be able to demonstrate the following in your field of study and also in a work context:

- knowledge and critical understanding of the well-established principles
- successful application of the range of knowledge and skills learned throughout your programme
- knowledge of the main methods of enquiry in your subject(s)
- the ability to evaluate critically the appropriateness of different approaches to problem solving
- effective communication of information, arguments and analysis, in a variety of forms, to specialist and non-specialist audiences
- qualities and transferable skills necessary for employment and progression to other qualifications requiring the exercise of personal responsibility and decision making
- the ability to utilise opportunities for lifelong learning, and should you wish to pursue it, a smooth transition route to an honours degree programme.

Your foundation degree will have been developed in line with relevant National Occupational Standards where appropriate. National Occupational

Standards recognise established benchmarks of competence. They are developed by employers, academics and other sector experts and define the skills and knowledge required to undertake particular job roles.

As competition for employment opportunities grows most foundation degrees offer a bridge between learning and earning. Authentic and innovative work-based learning is an integral part of a foundation degree. The work-based learning aspect of your foundation degree should offer you the opportunity of relevant work and training.

In your foundation degree, academic knowledge and understanding should integrate with, and support the development of, vocational skills and competencies. It should enhance and extend your career prospects and foster the development of life-long learning. You should get the opportunity to work on real projects, making a real difference whilst picking up technical and practical skills needed for your chosen career path.

Assessment

Different foundation degrees will assess your work in different ways. The purpose of assessment is to determine your performance in relation to the learning outcomes of your award, level and modules. Assessment methods will include a variety of formal and informal, summative and formative techniques. The assessment strategy for your programme is likely to provide a good mix of competency based assessments, examination and employer feedback that may include:

- case studies
- presentations
- project work
- examinations
- reports
- practicals or simulations
- observations and viva examinations
- peer and self assessment
- personal development plans and evidence portfolios.

You should understand the relationship between learning outcomes and assessment and develop your confidence in tackling different forms of assessment.

About BTEC Higher Nationals

BTEC Higher Nationals are designed to provide a specialist vocational programme, linked to professional body requirements and National Occupational Standards where appropriate. They offer a strong, sector-related emphasis on practical skills development alongside the development of requisite knowledge and understanding. The qualifications provide a thorough grounding in the key concepts and practical skills required in the sector and their national recognition by employers allows direct progression to employment. A key progression path for BTEC HNC and HND learners is to the second or third year of a degree or honours degree programme, depending on the match of the BTEC Higher National units to the degree programme in question

The BTEC HNC and HND in Sport and in Sport and Exercise Sciences offer progression routes to membership of The Institute of Sport and Recreation Management (ISRM) and The Institute for Sport, Parks and Leisure (ISPAL).

BTEC Higher Nationals in Sport and in Sport and Exercise Sciences have been developed to focus on:

- providing education and training for a range of careers in the sector
- the education and training of those who are employed, or aspire to be employed, in a variety of types of work, such as in performance analysis, nutrition for sport and exercise, sports therapy, sports development, sports coaching, education, research and development
- opportunities for you to gain a nationally-recognised vocationally-specific qualification to enter employment in the sector or progress to higher education qualifications such as a fulltime degree in a related area
- an understanding of the roles of those working in the sector, including how their role and that of their department fits within the overall structure of their organisation and within the community
- opportunities for you to focus on the development of the higher level skills in sport, sport and exercise sciences and related areas
- the development of your knowledge, understanding and skills in the field of sport, sport and exercise sciences and related areas
- opportunities for you to develop a range of skills, techniques and attributes essential for successful performance in working life.

Assessment

For BTEC Higher Nationals the purpose of assessment is to ensure that effective learning of the content of each unit has taken place. Evidence of this learning, or the application of the learning, is required for each unit. The assessment of the evidence relates directly to the assessment criteria for each unit, supported by the generic grade descriptors. The process of assessment can aid effective learning by seeking and interpreting evidence to decide the stage that you have reached in your learning, what further learning needs to take place and how best to do this. Therefore, the process of assessment should be part of the effective planning of teaching and learning by providing opportunities for both you and your assessor to obtain information about progress towards learning goals.

The role of the Sector Skills Councils

Sector Skills Councils (SSCs) are independent, employer-led, UK wide organisations that are licensed by government to build skills systems relevant to employment. They have four key goals:

- to reduce skills gaps and shortages
- to improve productivity, business and public service performance
- to increase opportunities for skills development
- to improve learning through National Occupational Standards, apprenticeships and further and higher education.

SSCs make labour market information available to key stake holders. This information is at the centre of effective careers counselling. SkillsActive is the SSC for Active Leisure, Learning and Wellbeing. This sector covers everything from the grass-roots through to performance sport and they ensure the sector has suitably qualified employees and volunteers to support the delivery of sport and sport related activities. Find out more about SkillsActive at www.skillsactive.com.

How to use this book

This book is divided into chapters that cover the theory you will need to help you through your studies and chapters that cover the practical aspects of studying for a foundation degree or a BTEC Higher National. This book contains many features that will help you use your skills and knowledge in work-related situations and assist you in getting the most from your course.

Features of this book

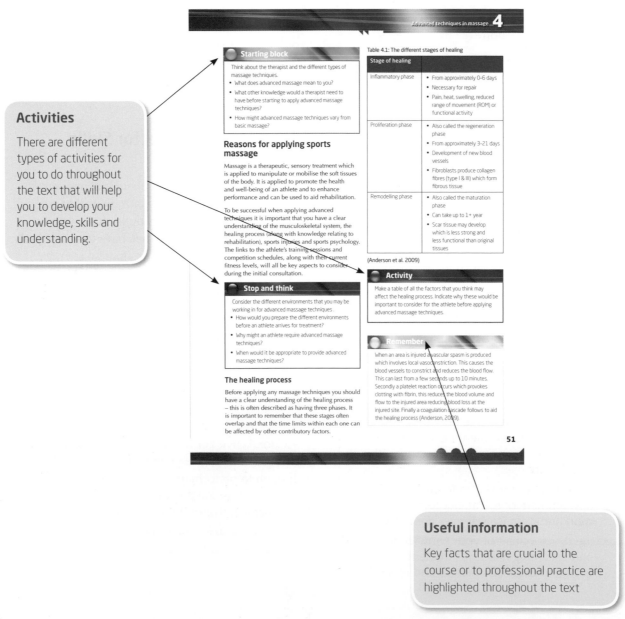

Activities

There are different types of activities for you to do throughout the text that will help you to develop your knowledge, skills and understanding.

Starting block

Think about the therapist and the different types of massage techniques.
- What does advanced massage mean to you?
- What other knowledge would a therapist need to have before starting to apply advanced massage techniques?
- How might advanced massage techniques vary from basic massage?

Reasons for applying sports massage

Massage is a therapeutic, sensory treatment which is applied to manipulate or mobilise the soft tissues of the body. It is applied to promote the health and well-being of an athlete and to enhance performance and can be used to aid rehabilitation.

To be successful when applying advanced techniques it is important that you have a clear understanding of the musculoskeletal system, the healing process (along with knowledge relating to rehabilitation), sports injuries and sports psychology. The links to the athlete's training sessions and competition schedules, along with their current fitness levels, will all be key aspects to consider during the initial consultation.

Stop and think

Consider the different environments that you may be working in for advanced massage techniques.
- How would you prepare the different environments before an athlete arrives for treatment?
- Why might an athlete require advanced massage techniques?
- When would it be appropriate to provide advanced massage techniques?

The healing process

Before applying any massage techniques you should have a clear understanding of the healing process – this is often described as having three phases. It is important to remember that these stages often overlap and that the time limits within each one can be affected by other contributory factors.

Table 4.1: The different stages of healing

Stage of healing	
Inflammatory phase	• From approximately 0–6 days • Necessary for repair • Pain, heat, swelling, reduced range of movement (ROM) or functional activity
Proliferation phase	• Also called the regeneration phase • From approximately 3–21 days • Development of new blood vessels • Fibroblasts produce collagen fibres (type I & III) which form fibrous tissue
Remodelling phase	• Also called the maturation phase • Can take up to 1+ year • Scar tissue may develop which is less strong and less functional than original tissues

(Anderson et al. 2009)

Activity

Make a table of all the factors that you think may affect the healing process. Indicate why these would be important to consider for the athlete before applying advanced massage techniques.

Remember

When an area is injured a vascular spasm is produced which involves local vasoconstriction. This causes the blood vessels to constrict and reduces the blood flow. This can last from a few seconds up to 10 minutes. Secondly a platelet reaction occurs which provokes clotting with fibrin, this reduces the blood volume and flow to the injured area reducing blood loss at the injured site. Finally a coagulation cascade follows to aid the healing process (Anderson, 2009).

Advanced techniques in massage 4

51

Useful information

Key facts that are crucial to the course or to professional practice are highlighted throughout the text

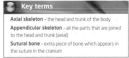

Functional anatomy **1**

Key structures of the skeletal system

The average adult skeleton consists of 206 bones. The precise number varies and with age some bones may become fused. The skeleton can be divided into two components: the **axial skeleton** contains 80 bones and the **appendicular skeleton** contains 126 bones.

> **Key terms**
>
> **Axial skeleton** – the head and trunk of the body
>
> **Appendicular skeleton** – all the parts that are joined to the head and trunk (axial)
>
> **Sutural bone** – extra piece of bone which appears in the suture in the cranium

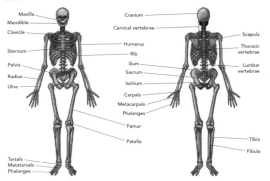

Figure 1.3: Bones of the skeleton

The number of bones can vary in the human body due to anatomical variation such as an extra lumbar vertebrae, cervical rib, lumbar rib or **sutural bones** in the skull. The appendicular skeleton is not fused, allowing for a much greater range of motion.

The axial skeleton (see Figure 1.4 a to c) forms the upright axis of the body and consists of the:

- cranium which consists of the parietal, temporal, frontal, occipital, ethmoid and sphenoid bones
- facial bones consisting of maxilla, zygomatic, mandible, nasal, palatine, inferior nasal concha, lacrimal and vomer bones

- hyoid bone which is a u-shaped bone located in the neck
- vertebral column consisting of the cervical, thoracic and lumbar vertebrae, as well as the sacrum and coccyx
- thoracic cage consisting of the sternum and ribs
- auditory ossicles consisting of the malleus, incus and stapes found in the inner ear.

5

Key terms

Technical words and phrases are easy to spot. You can also use the glossary at the back of the book.

Case studies

Case studies provide snapshots of real workplace issues and show how the skills and knowledge you develop during your course can help you in your career.

> **Case study**
>
>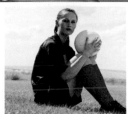
>
> Louise is representing her youth international football team and is in her second year at college. There is a major youth international tournament coming up and there has just been a change of coaching set-up in the team where a new manager and set of coaches have come in. Currently, Louise's father is suffering from testicular cancer and is in the early stages of treatment. Louise would normally be able talk to her partner about this but they have recently split up and this is playing on Louise's mind. Louise has started to worry a lot about how she is playing and training – and has started to worry that she may lose her place in the national team. During a game for her national team, Louise picks up an injury which means that she is going to be sidelined until one month before the tournament starts.
>
> 1. What are the different stressors and injury risk factors associated with this case?
> 2. What will some of Louise's responses to the injury be?
> 3. How could a sports therapist help Louise in this instance?
> 4. Would referrals to any other professionals be appropriate in this case?
> 5. How do you think Louise is going to react on her estimated return to sport, given how close it is to the international tournament?

Knowledge checks

At the end of each chapter these questions are there to check your knowledge. You can use them to see how much progress you've made and then check the answers on the companion website at **www.pearsonfe.co.uk/foundationsinsport**

> **Check your understanding**
>
> 1. How does the stress injury model of sports injury try to explain the causes of sports injury?
> 2. How can the attitudes of significant others increase the risk of sports injury?
> 3. What are the different models of responses to sports injury and how do they try to explain the psychological responses of injured athletes?
> 4. What signs should a sports therapist look for as indicators of poor adjustment to injury?
> 5. What are the typical behaviours of athletes who are adjusting to injury well and adhering to their programme correctly?
> 6. According to Heil (1993), what are the different stages in the rehabilitation of clients?
> 7. Why is social support a key factor in sports injury?
> 8. What does the acronym 'SMARTS' stand for and why is it important?
> 9. What are the benefits of using psychological skills training with injured athletes?
> 10. Name some of the different techniques used with injured athletes and discuss their benefits.

153

Chapter 1

Functional anatomy

Introduction

A comprehensive understanding of functional anatomy is essential for any good sports therapist. It can make the difference between passing or failing your foundation degree, or excelling within the industry. Understanding and knowing anatomical terms are fundamental to understanding medical notes and communicating with medical personnel. Anatomy can be learned through books and the Internet but there is no substitute for first-hand learning and application.

Functional anatomy is key to your ability to understand the assessment and diagnosis process, as well as providing sound clinical justification for treatment and rehabilitation. This chapter will help you to develop your understanding through the practical application of anatomy. It should be revisited frequently as you progress through the other chapters of the book. In a sports therapy foundation degree no module should be viewed in isolation. For example, while exploring *Chapter 3: Fundamentals of sports massage* identify the muscles you are working on. State their action, origin and insertion out loud. In *Chapter 5: Sports rehabilitation*, think about which muscles you are targeting, which joints are involved, what movements are occurring and the type of muscle contractions taking place.

Learning outcomes

After you have read this chapter you should be able to:

- understand anatomical terminology
- describe key structures of the skeletal system
- explain joint classifications
- describe key structures of the muscular system.

Anatomical terminology

Anatomical text is commonly used within the medical profession, in treatment notes and in communication between professionals. It is therefore very important you are able to understand the most common terms used. The anatomical position is the position your client assumes when you are documenting your anatomical terms (or the position your model assumes when demonstrating anatomical terms).

The anatomical position of a client is anteriorly viewed with arms by the side with forearms **supinated**. This is the position used for all anatomical references (see Figure 1.1). Table 1.1 describes common anatomical terminology used within sports therapy.

Three common anatomical terms used are sagittal, transverse and coronal planes.

Key term

Supinated – when the forearm is supinated the palm of the hand is facing forward when in the anatomical position

Sagittal plane – vertical plane (from head to toe) passing through the navel dividing the body into left and right.

Transverse plane – also known as the horizontal plane divides the body into superior and inferior body segments.

Coronal plane – also known as the frontal plane divides the body into dorsal and ventral segments (front and back).

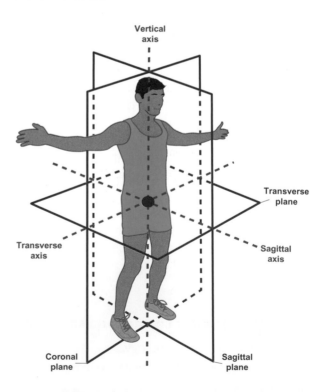

Figure 1.1: Planes

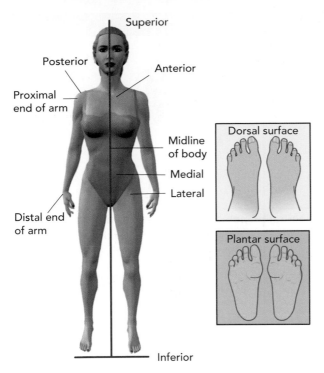

Figure 1.2: Anatomical positions

As a sports therapist you need to understand the movements available at each joint. Table 1.2 describes common movement terminology used in sports therapy. (Movements available at joints are addressed later in the chapter on page 13.)

Table 1.1: Anatomical terminology

Terminology	Description
Anterior	Front view, in front or towards the front of the body
Posterior	Rear view, behind or towards the rear of the body
Medial	Towards or at the midline of the body
Lateral	Away from or at the midline of the body
Proximal	Near to or closer to the centre of the body
Distal	Away from or further from the centre of the body
Superior	Above or towards the head of the body
Inferior	Below or away from the head of the body
Superficial	Nearer to the surface
Deep	Away from the surface
Ipsilateral	Same side as the body
Contralateral	Opposite side of the body
Prone	Lying face down
Supine	Lying face up

Table 1.2: Movement terminology

Movement	Description	Picture
Flexion	Reduction of the joint angle	
Extension	Increasing the joint angle	

Movement	Description	Picture
Abduction	Taking away from the midline	Abduction / Adduction / Circumduction
Adduction	Taking towards the midline	
Pronation	Palm turning downwards	Supination (radius and ulna are parallel) / Pronation (radius rotates over ulna) / Pronation / Supination
Supination	Palm turning upwards	
Plantarflexion	Pointing the toes away, pushing the sole of the foot away	Dorsiflexion / Plantar flexion
Dorsiflexion	Moving the top of the foot towards the body, showing the sole of the foot	
Hyperextension	Increased extension beyond the norm	Hyperextension / Extension / Flexion
Rotation	Movement of a bone (or the trunk) around its own longitudinal axis	Rotation / Lateral rotation / Medial rotation
Medial rotation	Turning towards the midline	
Lateral rotation	Turning away from the midline	

Key structures of the skeletal system

The average adult skeleton consists of 206 bones. The precise number varies and with age some bones may become fused. The skeleton can be divided into two components: the **axial skeleton** contains 80 bones and the **appendicular skeleton** contains 126 bones.

> ### Key terms
>
> **Axial skeleton** – the head and trunk of the body
>
> **Appendicular skeleton** – all the parts that are joined to the head and trunk (axial)
>
> **Sutural bone** – extra piece of bone which appears in the suture in the cranium

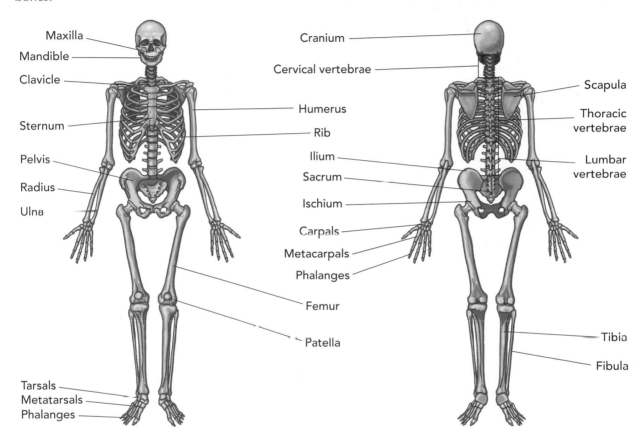

Figure 1.3: Bones of the skeleton

The number of bones can vary in the human body due to anatomical variation such as an extra lumbar vertebrae, cervical rib, lumbar rib or **sutural bones** in the skull. The appendicular skeleton is not fused, allowing for a much greater range of motion.

The axial skeleton (see Figure 1.4 a to c) forms the upright axis of the body and consists of the:

- cranium which consists of the parietal, temporal, frontal, occipital, ethmoid and sphenoid bones
- facial bones consisting of maxilla, zygomatic, mandible, nasal, palatine, inferior nasal concha, lacrimal and vomer bones

- hyoid bone which is a u-shaped bone located in the neck
- vertebral column consisting of the cervical, thoracic and lumbar vertebrae, as well as the sacrum and coccyx
- thoracic cage consisting of the sternum and ribs
- auditory ossicles consisting of the malleus, incus and stapes found in the inner ear.

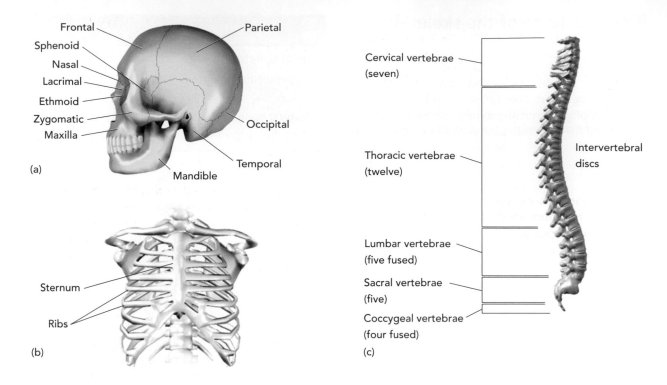

Figure 1.4: Bones of the axial skeleton: a) the cranium, b) the thorax, c) the vertebral column

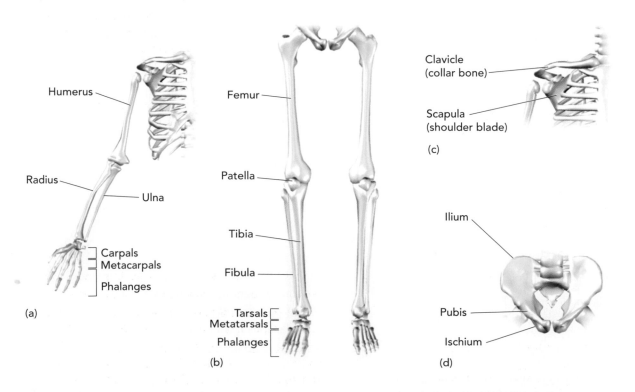

Figure 1.5: Bones of the appendicular skeleton: a) the upper limbs, b) the lower limbs, c) the shoulder girdle and d) the pelvis

The appendicular skeleton (Figure 1.5 a to d) consists of all the bones which attach to the axial skeleton, and can be divided into six regions.

- Each arm and forearm consists of humerus, ulna and radius.
- Each hand consists of 8 carpals, 5 metacarpals, 5 proximal phalanges, 4 middle phalanges, 5 distal phalanges and 2 sesamoid.
- Each pectoral girdle consists of 2 clavicle and 2 scapula.
- The pelvis consists of left and right os coxae, which are formed by the fusion of the illium, ischium and pubis.
- Each leg consists of a femur, tibia, patella and fibula.

Each foot contains 7 tarsals, 5 metatarsals, 5 proximal phalanges, 4 middle phalanges, 5 distal phalanges and 2 sesamoid bones.

Remember

Before you palpate structures on your model you must:
- ask and gain informed consent
- wash your hands thoroughly before and after. Antibacterial gel is a good substitute if you do not have washing facilities.

Activity

Using the diagrams above, palpate the bony landmarks listed below on your model:

- Mandible
- Clavicle
- Sternum
- Head of the humerus
- Distal part of the ulna
- Carpals bones
- Sacrum

- Ilium
- Distal parts of the femur
- Patella
- Distal part of the fibula
- Fifth metatarsal

Refer to Useful resources (page 20) and palpate the following:

- Acromion process
- Olecranon process
- Hook of hammate
- Medial border of scapula
- Anterior superior iliac crest (ASIS)
- Sustentaculum tali

- Posterior superior iliac crest (PSIS)
- L4
- Greater trochanter
- Lateral malleolus
- Calcaneus

Functions of the skeletal system

The skeletal system has a number of physiological and mechanical functions.

- **Protection** – the skeletal framework protects the vital tissues and organs in your body. The cranium protects the brain, the thorax protects the heart and lungs, the vertebral column protects the spinal cord and the pelvis protects the abdominal and reproductive organs.
- **Attachment for skeletal muscles** – the skeleton provides a framework for attachment of the skeletal muscles via tendons as well as the attachment of ligaments. The skeletal system provides a lever system in order to create joint motion and movement.
- **Support** – the skeletal frame provides a structural framework, giving the body a supportive framework for soft tissue, and providing shape.
- **Source of red blood cell production** – red bone marrow found within the bone produces red blood cells, white blood cells and platelets.
- **Store of minerals** – bone stores minerals such as calcium, phosphate (a stored form of phosphorus) and magnesium, which are essential for growth and bone health. Minerals are released into the bloodstream as the body requires them. The yellow bone marrow stores fat.

Remember

Functions of the skeleton can be remembered with the acronym PASSS.

Protection

Attachment

Support

Source

Storage

Male and female skeletal systems differ. A female pelvis is wider and flatter to assist childbirth, with associated widening of the sacrum. The cartilage found at the pubic symphysis in a female is broader allowing a greater spreading of the pelvis during childbirth. The female rib cage is more rounded and smaller than a male rib cage, with the lumbar curve greater and pelvis anteriorly tilted. The greater hip width results in an increased femur angle from the hip to the knee (increased Q angle). Males generally are taller and have heavier bones. Males have greater muscle bulk with tendon attachments being more prominent and easier to palpate.

Stop and think

The function of calcium is to promote healthy bone mass. Calcium also plays a vital role within exercise; an additional supply of calcium is required to ensure levels of calcium ions are adequate for working muscle to elicit the relaxatory response. Ninety nine per cent of calcium is found in bones and 1 per cent in the body's fluids and cells. A diet deficient in calcium can lead to osteopenia in later life. What kind of foods do you think contain calcium?

Types of bone

Bones are a specific shape and size for a reason.

Long bones (see Figure 1.6) such as the tibia, fibula, humerus and ulna are found in the limbs. They have a long shaft known as the **diaphysis**. Each end of the bone is known as the epiphysis.

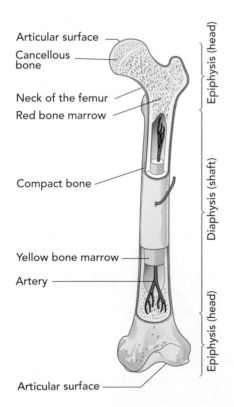

Articular surface
Cancellous bone
Neck of the femur
Red bone marrow
Compact bone
Yellow bone marrow
Artery

Epiphysis (head)
Diaphysis (shaft)
Epiphysis (head)

Articular surface

Figure 1.6: Structure of a long bone

- Short bones such as the carpals and tarsals (see Figure 1.5a, page 6) are found in the wrist and ankles. These are strong, small, light and cube shaped, consisting of cancellous bone encased by compact bone.
- Flat bones include the scapulae (see Figure 1.5c), sternum and bones of the cranium (see Figure 1.4a and b). They are thin, flat, have a large surface area and aspects curved in shape to allow for a strong attachment site. Flat bones are particularly strong and their function is to provide protection.
- Sesamoid bones such as the patella (see Figure 1.5b) are small bones located within a tendon.
- Irregular bones such as the vertebrae (see Figure 1.7) have irregular shapes and do not fit into any of the above categories.

The vertebral column

This is a segmented flexible pillar made up of five regions: the cervical, thoracic, lumbar, sacral and coccyx. Before the developmental years the vertebral column consists of 33 single vertebra. The cervical, thoracic and lumbar regions comprise a total of 24 single vertebra. During the developmental years five vertebrae fuse to form the sacrum, and between two and four fuse to form the coccyx.

The second cervical vertebra (C2) to the sacrum (S1) consists of individual **articulations**, held firmly in position by intevertebral discs (comprised of **fibrocartilage**) and ligaments. Due to the natural **lordosis** in the cervical and lumbar areas, the disc tends to be thicker **anteriorly**. Each vertebra consists of various processes, an arch and a body which supports the weight. The vertebral foramen is a hole through which the spinal cord passes (see Figure 1.7).

Key terms

Diaphysis – main shaft of the bone

Articulation – the contact of two or more bones at a specific location

Fibrocartilage – this cartilage is very rich in type 1 collagen and is strong and durable. It can be found, for example, in the menisci of the knee and intevertebral disc

Lordosis – exaggerated curvature of the lumbar spine

Anteriorly – towards the front

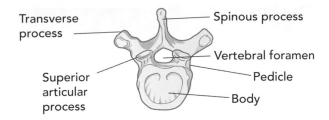

Figure 1.7: A vertebra

The movements available within each section of the vertebral column differ widely due to the complex anatomical structure. The vertebrae increase in size from the top down and are held together by strong ligaments, allowing minimal movement between individual vertebra, but allowing the vertebral column a considerable amount of flexibility. Generally, the degree of movement permitted reduces from top down. Gross movements of the vertebral column include flexion, extension, lateral flexion and rotation.

Stop and think

- The average vertebral column length is 72–75 cm.
- Intervertebral discs are responsible for 25 per cent of its length.
- The length of the vertebral column is responsible for 40 per cent of the height of the human.
- Age-associated decline in height is due to the thinning of the discs.

Your height can vary 2 cm during the day. This is **diurnal variation**. Measure yourself at the start and end of each day and compare the results.

The five regions of the vertebral column include:
- **Cervical section of the vertebrae** – this is the upper seven vertebrae (C1–C7) forming the cervical curve of the vertebral column in a convex shape. In functional anatomy the **occipital condyles** play an important function in transferring the weight of the head to C1. The first cervical vertebra (C1) is known as the **atlas**, and the second vertebra (C2) is known as the **axis** (its function is to rotate the head). The atlanto-occipital joint and atlanto-axial joint do not contain **intervertebral discs**. The joint type formed is a pivot joint, allowing movement of the cranium. The cervical vertebrae directly support

the weight of the head, and therefore have the most available movement, although stability is compromised. The cervical spine is further more vulnerable due to the vertebrae rising above the shoulders.

- **Thoracic section of the vertebrae** – the next 12 vertebrae (T1–T12) form the thoracic curve of the vertebral column in a concave shape. The peak of the thoracic curve is around T6–T8. The true ribs (first seven ribs) articulate directly with the sternum originating from the thoracic vertebrae to form the rib cage. Ribs eight to ten either 'float' or attach to the **costal cartilage**.
- **Lumbar section of the vertebrae** – the next five vertebrae (L1–L5). The lumbar region bears the largest portion of the body's weight, therefore the vertebrae are larger. L1–L5 are an important site for muscle attachment, in particular for the hip flexor (iliopsoas). L1–L5 form the lumbar curve of the vertebrae in a convex shape.
- **Sacral** – the sacrum is triangular in shape and articulates with the pelvis, and plays a significant role in absorbing the ground forces from the lower limb, and weight of the body above. The sacrum is formed from five fused vertebrae. The articulation between L5/S1 is known as the lumbosacral disc, while the articulation between the sacrum and coccyx forms the sacrococcygeal joint.
- **Coccyx** – the second fused section of the vertebrae consisting of approximately two to four vertebrae forms the remnants of the tail.

Key terms

Diurnal variations – fluctuations which occur each day

Occipital condyles – kidney-shaped with convex surfaces. There are two occipital condyles located either side of the foramen magnum. They articulate with the atlas bone

Intervertebral disc – a fibrocartilage disc which lies between each adjacent vertebrae of the spine

Costal cartilage – hyaline cartilage which connects the sternum to the ribs

The main functions of the vertebral column are to:

- encase and protect the spinal cord from injury
- distribute and absorb impact (the unique curvature and intervertebral discs act as a shock absorber)
- provide a surface for the attachment of the muscles which are responsible for moving the vertebrae, in turn maintaining balance and erectness of the trunk
- provide a surface for the attachment of the muscles of the pelvic girdle and pectoral area
- support the ribcage.

Whiplash injuries are a result of a violent collision propelling the neck into extension then flexion. The initial extension phase can result in posterior damage. In extreme cases superior vertebrae may dislocate, but more commonly cause damage to the restraining ligaments.

Activity

Using a variety of different models, observe the vertebrae, paying particular attention to:

- the cervical region (displays a convex curve (curved inwardly))
- the thoracic region (displays a concave curve (curved outwardly))
- the lumbar region (displays a convex curve (curved inwardly)).

Lordosis, kyphosis and scoliosis are acquired and congenital vertebral abnormalities. Over-exaggeration of the vertebral curves can hinder movement, affect muscular alignment, cause nerve compression, protruding or ruptured discs and possibly affect sporting performance.

Remember

Poor postural alignment can be caused by factors such as bone abnormalities and disease such as **ankylosing spondylitis**. These conditions should only be addressed by a medical practitioner or under medical guidance. If you are ever in doubt you should seek medical advice.

Key term

Ankylosing spondylitis – an inflammatory arthritis affecting mainly the joints in the spine and sacroilium in the pelvis. However, other joints of the body may also be affected as well as tissues including the heart, eyes, lungs and kidneys.

Lordosis

This is caused through an exaggeration of the lumbar curve, resulting in an increased anterior tilt of the pelvis. Muscular imbalances are inevitable, and may predispose the athlete to injury. Footballers presenting with exaggerated lumbar lordosis often present with associated muscle imbalances. Hamstrings present as lengthened and weak, whereas the opposing muscle group of the quadriceps present as shortened and strong. The incidence of hamstring injuries in football is high. However, Fijian/Polynesian athletes often present with exaggerated lumbar lordosis with no associated link to injury.

- Lengthened weak muscles include the hamstrings group and the abdominals. To correct the imbalance (if appropriate) lengthened weak muscles need to be strengthened with the use of exercises.
- Shortened strong muscles include the erector spinae and iliopsoas, rectus femoris, sartorius and tensor fascia latae. To correct the imbalance (if appropriate) shortened strong muscles should be lengthened through stretching or exercises such as yoga.

Kyphosis

This is caused through an exaggerated curve in the thoracic vertebrae. The scapulae are protracted, putting the scapulae and clavicles (shoulder girdle) under constant pull of gravity. Muscle balances are inevitable, and may predispose the athlete to upper body injuries.

- Lengthened weak muscles include the muscles responsible for scapular retraction and on the posterior aspect of the thoracic region such as trapezius and rhomboids. To correct the imbalance (if appropriate) lengthened weak muscles need to be strengthened with the use of exercises.

- Shortened strong muscles include anterior muscles of the thoracic region such as pectoralis major and minor. To correct the imbalance (if appropriate) shortened strong muscles should be lengthened through stretching or exercises such as yoga.

This condition is common in older people suffering from osteoporosis, osteoarthritis or can be congenital. If manipulated there is a risk of fracture.

Stop and think

Observe athletes' posture in a variety of sports. Do they present with a postural condition, e.g. lordosis or kyphosis? Why do they have this condition? Is it due to muscle imbalances which need correcting, or does their sport predispose them to this condition? Think of a skydiver, and the technique they assume in flight. You will observe most skydivers have lordosis. It would be detrimental to the athlete's performance if you attempted to correct this muscle imbalance.

Scoliosis

This can sometimes be observed or, on palpation of the vertebrae, an S or C shape can be felt deviating to the right or left.

- On observation of the spine, if the curve deviates to the left, muscles on the left aspect of the spine have shortened creating tension on the vertebrae to the left; the muscles on the right adapt by lengthening.

- If the curve deviates to the right then muscles on the right aspect of the spine have shortened creating tension on the vertebrae to the right; the muscles to the left adapt by lengthening.

Scoliosis is most commonly inherited and coexistent with pathology and developmental disorders such as cerebral palsy and cystic fibrosis. Upon observation you should refer to a medical practitioner for further advice if necessary.

Remember

If a postural condition is congenital then medical advice must be sought. However, if muscular imbalances are the fundamental cause then exercise therapy can be used in the correction.

To maintain correct posture the vertebrae should sit in neutral alignment. Many factors affect the *neutral* position of the vertebrae, for example, poor posture, injury, the sport played, incorrect exercise techniques, pregnancy, excess body composition (obesity), injury and disease. All of these can predispose the athlete to injury. It is important when performing exercise to consider safety at all times by ensuring a 'neutral spine alignment'.

Joint classifications

A joint is a junction where two or more bones articulate (meet). It plays a vital role in allowing movement to occur. Joints act as levers, allow movement and transmit and absorb forces. As a sports therapist you need a very good understanding of joints and their movement.

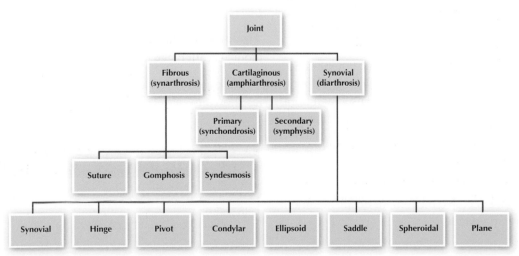

Figure 1.8: Types of joint

The **force transmission** as a result of sports participation can be excessive causing damage and requiring therapeutic intervention. *Chapter 10: Biomechanics of sports injury* will explore force transmission, biomechanics and associated sports injuries. Joints can be classified into three groups and each category can be further subdivided.

Synarthrosis/fibrous/fixed joints

The bones which articulate at fibrous joints are connected via fibrous connective tissue. They allow very limited movement. The three subcategories are:

- suture(s) – example = found between the cranial bones
- gomphosis (-es) – example = tooth in its socket
- syndesmosis (-es) – example = inferior tibiofibular joint.

Amphiarthrosis/cartilaginous/slightly moveable joints

The bones which articulate at cartilaginous joints are connected by either **articular (hyaline) cartilage** forming a primary joint such as first sternoclavicular joint, or fibrocartilage forming a secondary joint such as intervertebral disc, which may contain an internal cavity or nucleus. Movement permitted is greater than at fibrous joints.

Diarthrosis/synovial/freely moveable joints

Synovial joints allow a greater degree of movement than fibrous and cartilaginous. See Figure 1.9 for the structure of a synovial joint. Articular cartilage encases the end of bones that articulate at the joint, allowing freedom of movement and reduction of friction. The joint is surrounded by a strong fibrous capsule, which is lined with a synovial membrane (synovium) providing lubrication and nourishment to the articular cartilage. The **ligaments** attach bone to bone and further strengthen the fibrous capsule. Ligaments are located internal and external to the capsule, and further supported by the surrounding muscle attachments and strong **tendons**. Ligaments' function is to provide joint stability, thus preventing dislocation. If excessive movement occurs ligaments may become damaged.

Key terms

Force transmission – impact forces transmitted through the body

Articular cartilage – (also known as hyaline cartilage) is smooth and covers the surface of bones

Ligament – a band of tough fibrous tissue connecting bone to bone

Tendon – a band of inelastic tissue connecting a muscle to bone

Bursae are common features. They are fluid-filled sacs preventing friction between the sliding surfaces of structures such as ligaments, tendons and the capsule. Bursae are vulnerable to injury, resulting in a condition known as bursitis. The suffix 'itis' identifies inflammation is present. Bursitis is therefore inflammation of the bursa. Another common inflammatory condition is synovitis, inflammation of the synovial fluid or capsule.

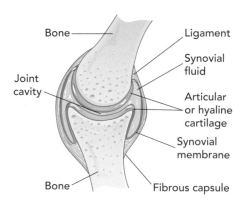

Figure 1.9: Structure of a synovial joint - transverse section of knee joint

Synovial joints can be subdivided into six categories as shown in Table 1.3.

Activity

Devise a table which has four columns labelled: Joint name; Joint type; Movements permitted; Sporting example. Complete the table for every joint.

Table 1.3: Subcategories of synovial joints

Joint name	Example	Movement	Figure
Hinge	Humero-ulnar joint	Flexion and extension	1
Pivot	Proximal radio ulnar joints	Rotation	2
Ellipsoid (condyloid)	Metacarpophalangeal	Flexion and extension Abduction and adduction	3
Saddle (sellar)	First carpometacarpal joint	Some rotation	4
Spheroidal (ball and socket)	Coxal joint	Flexion and extension Abduction and adduction Rotation	5
Plane (gliding)	Intercarpal joint	Sliding movements	6

Key structures of the muscular system

The human body contains three types of muscle tissue:

- skeletal such as gastrocnemius
- smooth which is found in the intestines
- cardiac which comprises the heart.

Skeletal tissue constitutes approximately 30–40 per cent of total human body mass, and is of great interest to sports therapists. It is vital you understand the function of skeletal muscle in relation to complex sporting movements.

Muscle tissue has two main functions: movement and posture.

- Production of movement: muscles are attached to the skeleton via a tendon or broad **aponeurosis**. When a muscle contracts, it exerts a force on the bone and produces movement. Muscles can pull but cannot push, and are positioned across joints in order to produce movement.
- Stabilisation of body positions: body positions are the result of skeletal contraction. Postural muscles contract continually to maintain body positions. The abdominal muscles help to stabilise the spine

when standing or sitting, while the erector spinae works to keep the spine erect.

Other functions of the muscular system include:

- assisting the movement of substances within the body such as blood, food, faeces, urine, gases and lymph
- **thermogenesis** – muscle contraction produces a by-product, heat, which helps maintain the normal body temperature of 37°C. Shivering, which is an involuntary contraction, can increase the rate of heat production considerably
- regulation of organ volume such as the stomach and bladder.

The muscular system contains over 640 named muscles. The main muscles relevant to a sports therapist can be seen in Figure 1.10.

As a sports therapist it is not enough just to learn the name and location of the muscles. You need to understand the action of each muscle. Muscle **origin** and **insertion** knowledge will assist the therapist in assessment, diagnosis, treatment and clinical justification. There are many resources which you can use to learn your origin and insertions, and in time progress to nerve innervations.

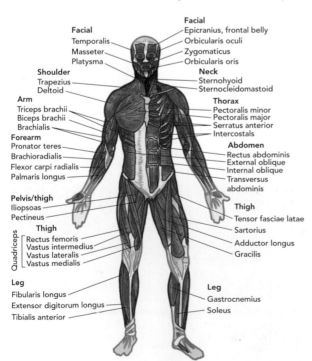

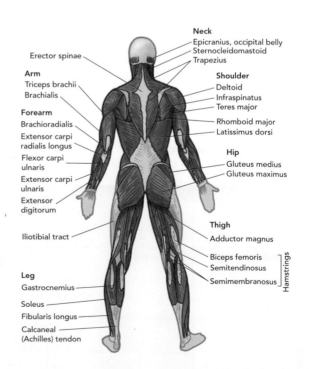

Figure 1.10: Anterior and posterior muscular system

Key terms

Aponeurosis – a flat, broad tendon

Thermogenesis – the process of heat production

Origin – the attachment site of a muscle to bone (in a few exceptions muscle). The origin is a fixed location

Insertion – the attachment of a muscle usually via a tendon to bone. The insertion on the bone is moveable as a result of muscle contraction

Properties of muscle

Muscle tissue has three main properties that enable the tissue to function optimally:

- excitability: it responds to stimuli (Excitability is the property of the neuromuscular junction to respond to a stimuli.)
- contractibility: it can contract forcefully when stimulated, resulting in isometric or isotonic contraction
- extensibility: it can stretch without tearing, and can contract forcefully after being stretched
- elasticity: after stretching or contracting it can return to its original length.

Gross muscle structure

A skeletal muscle consists of thousands of individual muscle fibres, encased by connective tissue called the **endomysium**. Individual muscle fibres are made up of muscle cells. Muscle fibres are bundled together into fascicles, around ten to 100 in any bundle, further encased by connective tissue called the **perimysium**. All the fascicles are collated together and encased by connective tissue called the **epimysium**, which surrounds the whole muscle. The endomysium, perimysium and epimysium all extend from the deep **fascia**.

Key terms

Endomysium – connective tissue encasing individual muscle fibres

Perimysium – connective tissue encasing fascicles

Epimysium – connective tissue which encases all the fascicles surrounding the whole muscle

Fascia – fibrous tissue binding together or separating muscles

Stop and think

The functional part of the muscle name generally represents its function, with the exception of the ankle. For example, a flexor decreases the angle at a joint bringing the anterior surfaces closer together (flexor carpi radialis main function is wrist flexion). Think about the following terms: extensor, adductor, supinator, pronator, levator and sphincter. Can you name a muscle and state its function for each term?

The endomysium, perimysium and epimysium are continuous connective tissue that may extend beyond the muscle tissue and form the tendon. The tendon is therefore a dense regular connective tissue. The Achilles tendon is a cord of dense connective tissue which is extended from the gastrocnemius, soleus and plantaris and attaches to the calcaneous. Extension of connective tissue from some muscles can be as a broad, flat layer known as an aponeurosis. The structure of the skeletal muscle is shown in Figure 1.11.

Activity

Using a resource such as the *Muscle Atlas* from the University of Washington's Department of Radiology (see *Useful resources*, page 20) draw up a table like the one below. Complete the table for each muscle. An example has been completed for you. This will provide a valuable resource for the rest of your sports therapy career.

Muscle	Action	Origin	Insertion	Nerve innervation
Biceps brachii	Supinates forearm, when supine flexes forearm	Short head: tip of coracoid process of scapula Long head: supraglenoid tubercle of scapula	Tuberosity of radius and fascia of forearm via bicipital aponeurosis	Musculocutaneous nerve (C5 and C6)

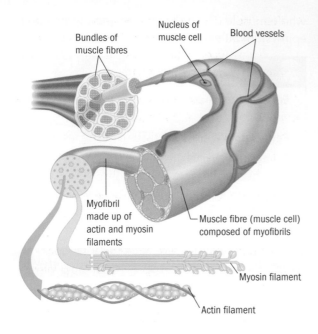

Figure 1.11: Organisation and structure of skeletal muscle

Superficial fascia separates muscle from the skin, provides protection, reduces heat loss and is storage for fat and water. Deep fascia holds similar functioned muscles together, facilitates free movement of muscles, blood vessels, lymphatic vessels, nerves and fills any gaps between muscles. Deep fascia divides muscles into compartments. For example, the lower leg is divided into four compartments by the deep fascia: anterior, lateral, posterior and deep posterior compartments.

The anterior compartment consists of the tibialis anterior, the extensor digitorum longus, and the extensor hallucus longus. Their function is to **dorsiflex** at the ankle. The tibialis anterior also **inverts** the foot.

The lateral compartment comprises the peroneus longus, peroneus brevis and peroneus tertius. Peroneus longus and brevis function is to **plantarflex** and **evert** the foot, while peroneus tertius dorsiflexes and everts the foot.

The posterior compartment comprises the gastrocnemius, soleus and plantaris. Their function is to plantarflex at the ankle. The gastrocnemius is the most superficial of the muscles and has two heads – lateral and medial. The soleus lies under the gastrocnemius and above the plantaris. All three insert into the Achilles tendon onto the calcaneous.

The deep posterior compartment comprises the tibialis posterior, flexor digitorum longus, and flexor hallucis longus. Their combined function is to aid plantarflexion. However, flexor hallucis longus also flexes the big toe, flexor digitorium longus flexes the rest of the toes and tibialis posterior inverts the foot. Remember that the posterior and deep posterior compartments all plantarflex at the ankle.

Micro muscle structure

In order to understand muscle contraction, you must understand the micro-structure of a muscle fibre. The cell membrane of the muscle fibre is known as the **sarcolemma**. A muscle fibre consists of long myofibrils (the length of the fibre) between which organelles such as mitochondria, glycogen granules and myoglobin are suspended in the sarcoplasm.

Myofibrils are the contractile elements, consisting of thin and thick myofilaments known respectively as actin and myosin (see Figure 1.11). The myofilaments do not run the length of the myofibril – they are organised into units called sarcomeres. Sarcomere units are repeated along the length of the myofibril, where actin and myosin are present in an overlapping formation.

Sliding filament theory

The sliding filament model of muscle contraction is a complex process. When a muscle receives a nerve impulse (stimulus) the lengths of actin and myosin (myofilaments) do not change, but are drawn closer together by sliding across each other forming cross bridges. The result is that the sarcomeres shorten due to the contraction of the myofibril. The myofibril becomes shorter and thicker, resulting in muscle contraction.

The relaxation phase is a passive process, where the cross bridges relax, actin and myosin return to their original position, thus the sarcomere and myofilament lengthen to their original position. The muscle relaxes.

The nerve impulse is based on the 'all or nothing law'. Each fibre is capable of either contracting or not contracting – there is no in between. The nerve impulse must reach a particular threshold to trigger the activation and stimulate the muscle fibres. Muscle fatigue occurs due to the inability to sustain the strength of contraction required.

Characteristics of muscle

The **fascicular arrangement** of a muscle affects the power and range of motion. The cross-sectional area of a muscle is the dependent factor for power output; a short fibre can contract as powerfully as a long fibre. A muscle fibre can shorten up to 70 per cent of its resting length upon contraction. Therefore, the greater the length of the fibres, the larger the range of motion produced. The arrangement of fascicles is dependent on the muscle function, and is generally structured to provide a compromise between power and range of motion. There are five fascicle arrangements of a muscle: parallel, fusiform, circular, triangular and pinnate (Figure 1.12).

1. **Parallel** – the fascicles are arranged parallel to the longitudinal axis of the muscle. The fascicles form a flat tendon at each end.

2. **Fusiform** – similar in structure to the parallel arrangement. However, the fascicles taper towards the tendons, resulting in the muscle belly being greater in diameter than the tendon attachments, e.g. biceps brachii. These muscles are limited in power.

3. **Circular** – the fascicles are in a circular arrangement. Sphincter muscles are circular and enclose an orifice (opening).

4. **Triangular** – the fascicles are spread over a broad area and taper into a thick tendon, which is central to the muscle belly. The appearance is that of a triangle, e.g. pectoralis major. Triangular arrangement often occurs where restrictive leverage is required.

5. **Pennate** – the tendon extends nearly the entire length of the muscle, with short fascicles. There are three types of pennate structure: unipennate, bipennate and multipennate.

Due to the short arrangement of fascicles, and the increased number of fibres in a smaller space, these muscles are very powerful.

- Unipennate – the fascicles are arranged on one side, e.g. extensor digitorium longus.
- Bipennate – the tendon is located centrally, with fascicles on each side, e.g. rectus femoris muscle.
- Multipennate – there are several tendons, with fascicles attached obliquely, e.g. deltoid muscle.

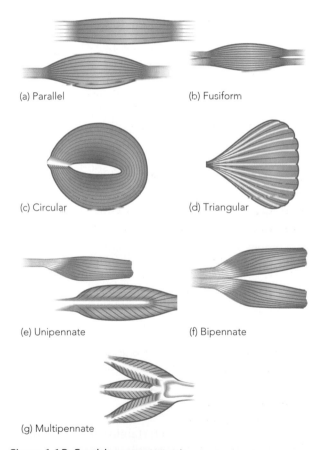

(a) Parallel

(b) Fusiform

(c) Circular

(d) Triangular

(e) Unipennate

(f) Bipennate

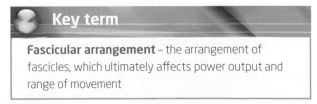

(g) Multipennate

Figure 1.12: Fascicle arrangement

Key term

Fascicular arrangement – the arrangement of fascicles, which ultimately affects power output and range of movement

Muscle attachments

Several muscles are used to produce effective movement. A high proportion of muscles have two attachments – an origin and insertion. However, there is a variety of muscles which have more than one origin and/or insertion. When the muscle receives a stimulus it contracts, attempting to bring the origin and insertion closer together. The contraction does not always result in muscle shortening. To achieve a wide variety of movements, muscles either work together or in opposition. To enable movement to occur, additional muscles are required to provide support and stabilisation. Skeletal muscles are referred to as **agonists**, **antagonists** and **synergists**.

Agonists are the prime movers producing the main movement, for example during knee extension the prime mover would be the quadriceps group. The hamstring group relax and lengthen allowing the knee to extend, referred to as the antagonist. However, when the hamstrings contract to produce knee flexion they become the agonist, while the antagonist (the quadricep group) relaxes to allow the movement to occur. Movements are rarely isolated, particularly during sport, therefore synergists and fixators play a major role.

Synergists are particularly important if the agonist muscles cross two joints to prevent any unwanted movement at the intermediate joint. For example, the biceps brachii crosses both the shoulder and elbow joint. Its primary action is on the forearm to provide flexion at the elbow. Synergists contracting at the shoulder prevent any unwanted movement. Synergist muscles may assist the agonist muscle in producing movement by altering the direction of pull to allow the most effective movement. During knee flexion the gastrocnemius and popliteus act as the main synergist.

Fixators are muscles which stabilise the origin of the agonist muscle, to allow the agonist to act more efficiently. The origin of the muscle is usually found at the proximal end of the limb which is stabilised by the fixators, while the movement occurs at the distal end where the muscle inserts.

Muscles are capable of performing contractile work in a variety of ways. Isotonic contractions result in the muscle creating movement such as concentric and eccentric contractions. Isometric contraction results in no movement.

- **Concentric contraction** – the muscle shortens as the tension in the muscle increases to overcome the opposing muscle (resistance), resulting in the muscle attachments moving closer together causing movement. The agonist muscle performs concentrically. During the elbow flexion phase of a bicep curl, the biceps and brachialis are the agonist muscle contracting concentrically.

- **Eccentric contraction** – the tension remains the same in the muscle. As the opposing force is greater the muscle lengthens. The antagonist muscle performs eccentrically. During elbow flexion the triceps contract eccentrically. Eccentric contraction is important in slowing down and controlling movement, which would otherwise be rapid due to gravity.

- **Isometric contraction** – the tension within the muscle increases, although the length of the muscle does not alter, thus no movement is created. If the bicep curl is held in mid range the muscles perform isometrically. The muscles do not change in their length, but support the weight.

Key terms

Agonist – the muscle producing the action (movement)

Antagonist – the muscle opposing the action (movement)

Synergist – synergist muscles assist the agonist muscles and provide stabilisation to prevent any unwanted movement

Fixator – provide stabilisation at the proximal end of the limb

Concentric – muscle contraction generates force which causes muscle shortening

Eccentric – the muscle lengthens due to the opposing force being greater than the force generated by the muscle

Isometric – force is generated by the muscle without changing length

Remember

Eccentric contractions are interesting to sports therapists. Athletes whose sports involve a high proportion of eccentric contraction are predisposed to injuries such as muscle tears and damage to the connective tissue. Eccentric exercises are useful in prehabilitation and rehabilitation programmes.

Case study

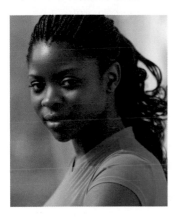

Jo Lee is a triathlete and has recently had her most victorious triathlon yet. The sprint triathlon consisted of a 400 m swim, 20 km on the bike followed by a 5 km run. Jo achieved an overall time of 1 hour 11 minutes 21 seconds, finishing second in the 25–29 years age group and an overall ranking of thirteenth female. Jo's swim split was impressive – fastest lady with 6 minutes 4 seconds positioning her seventh fastest overall of all male and female competitors and age groups. With a modest ride on the bike with a split of 41 minutes 12 seconds and a 5 km run in 21 minutes 30 seconds, Jo's training regime requires commitment and dedication consisting of 3 swim sessions a week (1 x 2 hours, 2 x 1 hour), 4 run sessions (3–9 miles per run, with a mixture of speed, interval and endurance), and 4 bike sessions covering around 8 miles each session with a longer weekly ride around 20–30 miles. In addition to this, 1 x 1 hour circuits, 1 x 1 hour pilates and one other session such as body balance or core weekly with a fortnightly 1 x 1 hour spin session.

1. Discuss the joint movements involved in front crawl swimming.
2. Discuss the muscles responsible for the movements identified in question 1.
3. Discuss the joint movements involved in cycling.
4. Discuss the types of muscle contraction occurring for movements identified in question 3.

Check your understanding

1. Describe the axial and appendicular skeleton, making reference to the names, types of bones and their function.
2. Palpate the following bony prominences on a client:
   - acromion process
   - spine of the scapula
   - sternoclavicular joint
   - L4 (lumbar vertebrae 4)
   - ischial tuberosity
   - third phalanges
   - posterior superior iliac crest (PSIS)
   - anterior superior iliac crest (ASIS)
   - sacroiliac joint
   - calcaneus
3. Briefly describe the three classifications of joints.
4. Describe the gross and micro-structure of a muscle
5. Differentiate between the functions of a ligament and a tendon.
6. Describe lordosis and its effect on the muscular system.
7. Describe kyphosis and explain which sports may predispose an athlete to this condition.
8. Observe a rugby player performing a squat and complete the following table for the up and down phase.

Agonist muscle	Action	Origin	Insertion

To obtain answers to these questions visit the companion website at www.pearsonfe.co.uk/foundationsinsport

Useful resources

To obtain a secure link to the websites below, see the Websites section on page ii or visit the companion website at www.pearsonfe.co.uk/foundationsinsport.

Muscle Atlas from the University of Washington Department of Radiology

Instant Anatomy

Visible Body

BBC Science Human Body

Get Body Smart Muscular Systems

Anatomy images from Imaios

Virtual Body from MEDtropolis

List of links to interactive anatomy resources from Class Brain

The following are also useful resources:

Gray's Anatomy for Students Flash Cards

Netter's Anatomy Flash Cards

Further reading

Agur, A. and Dalley, A. (2009). *Grants Atlas of Anatomy* 12th Edition. Philadelphia: Lippincott, Williams & Wilkins.

Behnke, R. (2001). *Kinetic Anatomy*. Champaign: Human Kinetics.

Field, D. and Hutchinson, J. (2006). *Anatomy, Palpation and Surface Markings*. London: Elsevier.

Harris, P. and Ranson, C. (2008). *Atlas of Living and Surface Anatomy for Sports Medicine*. China: Churchill Livingstone

Jarmey, C. (2008). *The Concise Book of Muscles*. Chichester: Lotus.

Kingston, B. (2005). *Understanding Muscles. A Practical Guide to Muscle Function* 2nd Edition. Cheltenham: Nelson Thornes.

Kingston, B. (2000). *Understanding Joints. A Practical Guide to Their Structure and Function*. Cheltenham: Nelson Thornes.

Manocchia, P. (2007). *Anatomy of Exercise*. London: A & C Black.

Palastanga, N., Field, D. and Soames, R. (2006). *Anatomy and Human Movement* 5th Edition. London: Elsevier.

Seeley, R., Stephens, T. and Tate, P. (2007). *Anatomy and Physiology*. Maidenhead: McGraw-Hill.

Standring, S. (2008). *Gray's Anatomy: The Anatomical Basis of Clinical Practice, Expert Consult* (online and print). Churchill-Livingstone.

Tortora, G.J. and Grabowski, S.R. (2000). *Principles of Anatomy and Physiology* 9th Edition. New York: John Wiley & Sons.

Wirhed, R. (2006). *Athletic Ability and the Anatomy of Motion* 3rd Edition. China: Mosby.

Chapter 2

Introduction to sports injury and assessment

Introduction

Regular participation in sport and exercise has positive physical, mental and social health enhancing properties. These include improved quality of life and vigour, reduced risk of chronic disease such as cardiovascular disease (CVD), diabetes, obesity, and depression, improved longevity and the maintenance of independence into older age.

However, regular participation in sport and exercise can sometimes have a detrimental effect on health in the form of injury. The effects that such injuries have on an individual's health can be relatively minor, with only a short period of rest needed, or more profound resulting in athletes having to retire from their careers. Sport- and exercise-related injuries do not just affect elite performers, but are a significant problem at every level of participation. Around a third of all emergency consultations are directly linked to sport and exercise. Although participation in any form of activity carries a risk of injury the overall health benefit of activity far outweighs this risk.

Learning outcomes

After you have read this chapter you should be able to:

- define sports injury
- classify sports injuries
- understand common causes of sports injuries
- understand how to prevent sports injuries
- identify common sport-related injuries
- understand how the body reacts to being injured
- explain key principles of sports injury assessment.

You have been appointed as the sports therapist for a professional rugby league club. The head coach you will be working with mentions that over the last few seasons the club has been suffering with high occurrence of injury. He would like you to reduce the number of injuries his players get. Consider the following:

- How you would approach this task?
- What information will you need to gather?

Definitions of sports injury

Sport injuries are diverse in terms of the mechanism of injury, how they present in individuals, and how the injury should be managed. Defining exactly what a sports injury is can be problematic and definitions are not consistent. In this chapter a sports injury is defined as any damage to tissues as a direct result of participating in sport and exercise, which causes the frequency and/or intensity of participation to be changed or ceased. This definition includes minor sports injuries that may not receive medical treatment in addition to more severe injuries that do require medical attention.

All sports injuries can be sustained in a normal active lifestyle. For example, a grade II sprain of the ankle can be sustained as a result of a poor tackle in soccer, or by stumbling on a poorly maintained footpath while out walking.

Occurrence of sports injuries

Sports injuries are common. However, it is difficult to answer the following questions:

- Which are the most dangerous sports?
- Do most injuries occur in training or competition?
- Which are the most common injuries across sports?

To be able to answer these questions reliably, the terms 'incidence' or 'prevalence' are used.

Incidence describes the rate of injuries in a given time frame, in a given population. It is usually expressed as new injuries sustained per 1000 hours of participation time. For example, if a marathon runner trains for 52 weeks of the year at 10 hours per week, this gives them an injury exposure time of 520 hours. If they sustain 5 injuries in this time frame the incidence is 9.62 injuries per 1000 hours participation (5 ÷ 520 x 1000).

The incidence calculation can also be used to accurately inform of injuries in training versus competition, across levels of participation (Bronner, Ojofeitimi and Mayers, 2006). It can also be used to look at specific injuries, for example, anterior cruciate ligament (ACL) sprains in skiing. Looking at sports injury incidence allows like-for-like injury comparison across sports without participation rate bias. Soccer carries the highest risk of sport injury because more people participate in this sport (Bahr and Mæhlum, 2004).

Stop and think

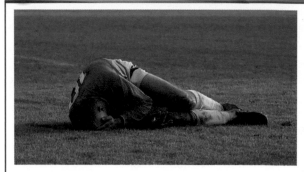

A team of 16 soccer players trains for 8 hours a week during a 40-week season. If the team sustains 46 injuries, what is the incidence of injury?

The term **prevalence** describes the percentage of athletes in a given population that have a sports injury at a given time. For example if you were working with a tennis club and 5 out of the 50 club players reported lateral elbow pain the prevalence would be 10 per cent. The term incidence is best suited to describing acute injuries, while prevalence is best suited to describe occurrence of overuse injuries.

Classification of sports injuries

There are many ways to classify sports injuries based on the time taken for the tissues to become injured, tissue type affected, severity of the injury, and which injury the individual presents with.

Acute versus overuse

This is one of the most common methods of classifying sports injuries, and relies on the sports therapist knowing the mechanism of injury and the onset of the symptoms. Acute injuries occur due to sudden trauma to the tissue, with the symptoms of acute injuries presenting themselves almost immediately. These are the injuries that most of us have seen while watching sport and a player requires medical attention. An example of an acute injury is a hamstring strain in 100 metre sprinting. Common acute injuries include:

- sprains
- strains
- fractures
- dislocations.

Overuse injuries are not so pervasive and represent a greater challenge to a sports therapist in diagnosis and management (Brukner and Khan, 2006). Overuse injuries occur over a period of time, usually due to repetitive loading of the tissue, with symptoms presenting gradually. For example, an overuse injury common to marathon runners is illiotibial band (ITB) syndrome (Fredericson and Wolf, 2005). In contrast to acute injuries, the cause of overuse injuries is much less obvious. Common overuse injuries include:

- patello femoral joint dysfunction
- medial tibial stress syndrome
- iliotibial band syndrome

Distinguishing between overuse and acute injuries can be difficult. For example, delayed onset muscle soreness (DOMS) and blisters are overuse injuries due to the mechanism of injury, although their symptoms present relatively quickly.

Tissue type

Sports injuries can be classified according to which tissue has become damaged. This allows sports therapists to identify soft, hard, and special tissue injuries. On occasion however, a sports injury can damage more than one tissue type, for example, a poor tackle in soccer could lead to an open fracture affecting all tissue types (see Table 2.1).

Table 2.1: The different types of tissue injury and examples of anatomical structures

Tissue type	Examples
Soft	muscle ligament tendon skin deep fascia fibrocartilage
Hard	bone joints articular cartilage
Special	brain peripheral nerves eyes nose sinuses organs teeth blood vessels

Using this classification method shown in Table 2.1 clasify:

- a muscle strain is a soft tissue injury
- a fracture is a hard tissue injury
- a concussion is a special tissue injury.

Severity

Most sports injuries require a period of time where participation is reduced or ceased due to symptoms. Therefore sports injuries can also be classified relating to how long the symptoms present themselves for. This classification method allows a sports therapist to describe injuries as mild, moderate, and severe:

- Mild injuries usually last for 1–7 days, and include haematoma (see Figure 2.1), blisters, and DOMS.
- Moderate injuries usually last for 8–20 days, and include low-grade muscle strains and ligaments sprains.
- Severe injuries usually last for 21 days but can lead to permanent damage. Examples of severe injures are fractures and high grade strains and sprains.

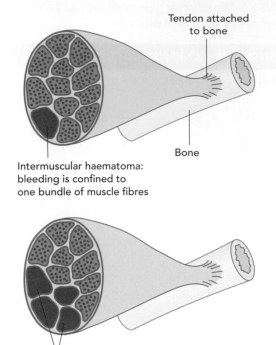

Tendon attached to bone

Bone

Intermuscular haematoma: bleeding is confined to one bundle of muscle fibres

Intramuscular haematoma: bleeding has spread to several bundles of muscle fibres

Figure 2.1: Types of haematoma

Primary consequential versus secondary non-consequential

An individual may sustain further injury as a result of being injured. An individual could get lower back pain due to the change of posture caused by limping because of a lateral collateral ligament (LCL) sprain (see Lewis, Schwellnus and Sole (2000) for more information on the aetiology and clinical features of low back pain in distance runners). In this example, the primary injury is the LCL sprain. The lower back pain was caused as a result of the original injury, so it is the secondary injury. A sports therapist can reduce the occurrence of secondary injury by:

- promoting good posture and gait
- carefully planning rehabilitation programmes and goals
- not allowing individuals to return to sport before the tissues are fully healed
- correctly adjusting crutches and fitting of braces and tape.

See Emery, Rose, McAllister and Meeuwisse (2007) and Kroll, Neri and Ho (2007) for examples of injury prevention strategies.

Common causes of sports injuries

To be able to effectively diagnose, rehabilitate, and ultimately prevent subsequent injury a sports therapist should understand the **aetiology** of the sports injury.

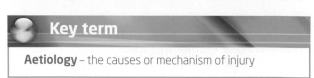

Key term

Aetiology – the causes or mechanism of injury

Identifying the exact cause of an injury can represent a significant challenge as the aetiology is not always obvious. The same injury sustained in two different individuals can also have completely different aetiology. For example, ITB syndrome could be caused by inappropriate footwear for participation or excessive downhill running or a leg length discrepancy. Finding the cause of a sports injury requires you to have detailed understanding of:

- the physical demands of the sport/exercise
- the psychological demands of the sport/exercise
- the appropriate equipment that should be used
- the surface of competition and/or training
- the individual's training: frequency, intensity, duration, and type.

Essentially sports injuries are caused by intrinsic factors and extrinsic factors (Baher and Holme, 2003).

Key intrinsic causes of sports injury

An intrinsic factor relates to the individual's inherent internal anatomical and pathological make-up.

Key extrinsic causes of sports injury

An extrinsic factor relates to various external or environmental factors relating to training/competition such as equipment, facilities or training methods.

Table 2.2: Intrinsic cause of injury

Anatomical factors	Relate to the make-up of the body. Leg length differences and body misalignment can lead to unequal forces being transferred to the tissues of the ankle, knee, hip, and back. An excessive quadriceps angle (Q-angle) can put strain on the ligaments of ankle and knee joints. Laxity of joints can lead to unnatural and often harmful movement leading to injury. Be aware that the laxity of a female's joints can increase when she is pregnant.
Physiological factors	Relate to how the body operates and facilitates movement. Injury can occur due to early onset of fatigue when a fatigued muscle cannot produce the same power and speed as a non-fatigued muscle even though the physiological demands placed upon it may not change. Reduced flexibility can lead to tight muscles that when overstretched exceed their ability and strain. Hyper-flexibility can allow harmful movements such as hyperextension. Muscle weakness or imbalance can lead to a discrepancy between agonist and antagonist in sporting movements and can place excessive strain on the body's soft tissue.
Individual difference factors	Specific to each individual and their medical history. Previous injuries and conditions can make a person more at risk of injury: tissues may not have healed effectively or returned to a non-damaged state. For example, ligament injuries; some athletes have a recurrent sprain in the same ankle or knee throughout their career.
Age factors	As the body ages it alters: less able to produce force, recovers slower, and soft tissues lose ability to stretch. An ageing body with demands of sport/exercise placed upon it can fail. A young, growing body can also be at risk of injury as tissues develop at different rates and cannot withstand strain placed upon them. For example overuse injuries are common in young athletes for this reason, e.g. shin splints and Osgood-Schlatter disease.

Table 2.3: Extrinsic cause of injury

Training-related factors	Relate to design of training programmes. Excessive repetitive loading of the tissues is needed for successful adaptation, however, without suitable recovery, tissues never have the chance to adapt and can fail. Sudden increase in frequency, intensity and duration, or simply changing training method can go beyond the tissues fail tolerance level leading to increased risk of injury. Performing techniques poorly can also place excessive strain on tissues. For example, poor shot technique in tennis increases the risk of tennis elbow.
Equipment selection factors	Relate to the suitability of equipment. Incorrect footwear will not protect the foot and ankle adequately nor distribute forces effectively, leading to an increased risk of injury. Not adhering to PPE rules place individuals under increased risk of injury. Training or competing with equipment that is not the correct size or weight can make movements biomechanically inefficient and put tissues under strain.
Environmental factors	Include environmental temperature and the surface participation takes place on. Surfaces that are too hard or too soft can lead to excessive forces going through the body or lead to a greater risk of sprains, e.g. feet/legs stuck in wet turf. Uneven surfaces, such as cambered paths or roads, can increase forces placed through one side of the body.
Psychological factors	Relate to the psychological demands of training/competition and how individuals respond to these demands. Being over- or under-aroused can lead to poor decision making and possible injury. When competing individuals can become over assertive or aggressive which can lead to them harming themselves or others. See *Chapter 12: Psychology of sports injuries* for more information.
Nutritional factors	Include adequate glycogen stores, hydration and protein intake. Adequate glycogen stores reduce the time taken to become fatigued. Correct hydration reduces the effect of dehydration, prevents **hyponatremia** and overheating of the body. Without correct protein intake, an individual's soft tissue may not recover or adapt properly, and can lead to DOMS and overtraining syndrome.

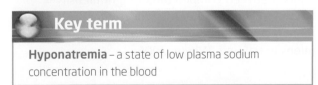

Key term

Hyponatremia – a state of low plasma sodium concentration in the blood

More often than not a sports injury is the result of a number of inter-related factors. Intrinsic factors can lead to a predisposition to sports injury that when combined with exposure to extrinsic factors leads to sports injury. Figure 2.2 below explains how sports injuries could be caused.

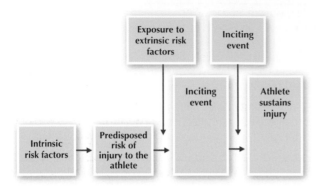

Figure 2.2: Injury aetiology and mechanism model demonstrating how intrinsic and extrinsic risk factors contribute to sports injury. (Adapted from Meeuwisse (1994))

Preventing sports injuries

One of the most important roles of sports therapists is preventing sports injuries and the physical, mental, social and financial harm that accompanies them. Primary preventative measures aim to reduce the occurrence of any injury within a sport/exercise. Secondary preventative measures relate to the sports therapist examining the injured athlete to work out how to reduce the risk of subsequent or secondary injuries. Any approach to preventing injury in an individual or team context should be sequential and follow the stages as shown in Figure 2.3 below.

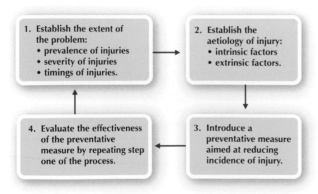

Figure 2.3: The sequential approach to preventing sports injury

There are general preventative measures that a sports therapist can use: they should be applied to the specific sport or exercise the individual participates in. For example, the personal protective equipment needed in boxing is completely different from that needed in soccer.

Warm-up and cool-down

A well-structured warm-up and cool-down is necessary to either prepare the individual physically and mentally or aid recovery from sport/exercise.

A good warm-up:

- increases blood and nutrient flow to the muscles
- improves neuromuscular functioning
- disperses **synovial fluid** across joints aiding movement
- mirrors sport-specific movements
- increases concentration.

A good cool-down:

- promotes **venous return**
- lactate removal
- improves flexibility
- improves relaxation.

Key terms

Synovial fluid – fluid within synovial joints that lubricates the joint

Venous return – the flow of blood back to the heart

Plyometric – a form of power training that involves eccentric actions followed by rapid concentric actions

Planning a session

You should plan any training or rehabilitation programme carefully considering frequency, intensity, duration, and type of training method. If programmes are carefully periodised it allows a gradual specific adaptation to imposed demands (SAID) and reduces damage to the tissues as a result of training (Whyte, 2006). Planned active or passive recovery allows tissue to repair themselves without injury. Between competition or high-intensity training such as **plyometric** work, individuals need more recovery in comparison to low-moderate intensity training (Whyte, 2006).

Training and competition should take place on an appropriate surface that allows for the demands of the sport to be met and reduces the forces going through the body. A risk assessment should be conducted on all training environments to identify risk and hazards and look to reduce these. For more details of how to conduct a risk assessment see *Chapter 12: Ethics and safety*. A technical observation of athletes to ensure skills/techniques are performed safely and effectively will also reduce injury risk. *Chapter 7: Training and conditioning* discusses training programme design in more detail.

Protective equipment

The use of protective equipment varies across different sports and exercises. The general purpose of protective equipment is to prevent harmful movements, reduce or disperse shock and force, and act as a shield to block force. Key pieces of protective equipment are footwear, helmets, goggles, gum shields, shin pads, gloves, bindings, and shoulder pads. It is common for athletes who have been previously injured to require bracing or taping of joints as an important secondary preventative measure to restrict harmful movements.

Adherence to the rules

If all performers are aware of and adhere to the rules and laws of the game then injuries can be reduced. This means that aggressor and victim will hopefully not sustain injury. Individuals should be coached in the differences between assertion and aggression to limit injuries.

Regular fitness testing

All participants in a sport should be able meet the demands of that sport or exercise. Individuals must be fit enough to train or compete, otherwise their tissues can fail. Regular fitness testing will ensure individuals have the basic fitness to participate safely and effectively. The use of field-based and laboratory-based testing can highlight any weaknesses in individuals that may lead to injury.

Psychological training

Some form of mental skills training and practice could reduce injury by reducing anxiety, improving attentional focus and allowing an athlete to achieve optimal arousal for their sport. *Chapter 11: Psychology of Sports Injury* discusses psychological training in more detail.

Meeting nutritional requirements

Active individuals have increased nutritional requirements to meet extra energy, hydration and recovery needs. Increasing carbohydrate, fluid, and protein intake can play an important role in injury prevention by delaying fatigue and promoting recovery. Certain supplements can promote recovery and maintain joint health, however, their value needs further empirical evidence (Goggs et al., 2005).

Common causes of sports injuries

There are a number of common sports injuries where a full understanding will help you to become a more effective professional. Each sport has its own common injuries and they are largely based on the physical demands of the sport. For example, in a sport like basketball where explosive movements and sudden changes in direction are needed, strains and sprains are common (Starkey, 2000). Table 2.4 explains key sports injuries.

Stop and think

Look at Table 2.4 to answer the following questions.
- Which do you think are overuse injuries and which are acute injuries, and why?
- Which injuries do you think require hospital treatment, and why?

Table 2.4: Common sport- and exercise-related injuries

Sports injury	Description	Likely aetiology
Haematoma	Bleeding under the skin or bruising. Can occur within muscle (intramuscular) or between the tissues (intermuscular).	Most likely caused by a direct blow damaging the blood vessels in a local area.
Strain	Tearing of muscle fibres with pain, swelling and loss of muscle strength evident. Graded I–III based on severity of symptoms and fibres torn; Grade III is a complete tear of the muscle.	Muscle fibres fail to cope with the demands placed upon them. Muscle are likely to tear via overstretching, or rapid acceleration/deceleration.
Sprain	A partial or complete tear of a ligament with symptoms of pain, swelling, bruising, loss of function, and often an audible 'popping sound'. They are graded I–III based on number of fibres torn; Grade III is a total rupture.	Usually caused by a direct trauma to a joint such as a tackle. Can be caused indirectly by twisting or falling in the absence of a blow or collision.
Fracture	A crack or full break in bone/s. Can be closed or open where the bone punctures the skin. Have symptoms of intense pain, loss of function, swelling, bruising, and possible deformity.	Caused by direct trauma such as a blow, or indirect trauma such as falling and breaking the fall with the wrist.
Dislocation	Partial (subluxation) or total (luxation) separation of a joint. Most commonly affects ball and socket joints. Symptoms include pain, bruising, swelling, loss of function, and deformity.	Caused by a direct blow or trauma which forces the joint to separate.
Concussion	A head injury with a temporary loss of brain function, concussion can cause a variety of physical, cognitive, and emotional symptoms.	Caused by a direct blow or collision to the head.
Contusions	Local muscle damage and bleeding with accompanying swelling and pain. Contusion to anterior thigh is known as a 'dead leg'.	Usually a direct blow from an opponent or contact with equipment in collision.
Tendinopathy	Refers to a range of tendon injuries with associated local pain upon movement. Common sites are patella, rotator cuff, wrist flexor, and Achilles tendons.	Excessive repetitive use of joints such as jumping, running, and throwing.
Bursitis	Inflammation of the bursa, usually in shoulder, hip, and heel. Symptoms of local tenderness, pain, and swelling are common.	Usually associated with overuse of joints, however can be caused by trauma to a joint. Can be a common secondary injury.
Plantar fasciitis	Pain, and sometimes inflammation of the plantar fascia (underside of the foot) which support the foot arch.	Usually caused by repetitive running-based training on hard ground, poor footwear, and poor foot biomechanics.
Stress fracture	A microfracture in bone, usually tibia, leading to localised pain and tenderness.	Excessive overload stress caused by large impact forces or repetitive action of muscles pulling across the bone.
ITB syndrome	Tightness of the ITB leading to pain which can be located from hip to lateral knee. Often made worse by running or eccentric activities such as walking down stairs.	Usually caused by repetitive use of quadriceps muscles without adequate rest. Other causes are the use of poor footwear on hard ground, biomechanical inefficiencies such as pronation, and hill running.
DOMS	Muscle soreness developing 24–48 hours after exertion. Symptoms are more severe after eccentric exercise.	Excessive overloading and over-reaching during training and competition.

How the body reacts to injury

The inflammatory process is the body's response to being injured. The inflammatory process has three main stages: the inflammatory stage, the proliferative phase and the maturation phase.

The inflammatory stage

This stage lasts for three to five days. Inflammation is a local response to cell damage within a tissue and is a chain of events that helps the body to repair, re-form, or form new scar tissue. Inflammation from sports injuries can be caused by excess pressure, friction, overload, over-stretching or impact trauma. There are five main signs and symptoms:

1. **Pain:** due to an increase in pressure in the injured area and damage that has been caused to local nerve fibres (nociceptors) from the swelling

2. **Swelling:** due to the bleeding from torn blood vessels and tissue fluid leaving the cells surrounding the injury

3. **Redness or discoloration:** due to the **vasodilation** of nearby undamaged blood vessels

4. **Heat:** due to the dilation of blood vessels, and thus local area circulation, around the injury site

5. **Loss of function:** due to the pain and swelling caused by the injury. Function maybe reduced or lost totally, including the inability to bear any weight on injured limbs.

The signs and symptoms of inflammation are related to the degree of injury. The higher the degree of injury, the greater the signs and symptoms of

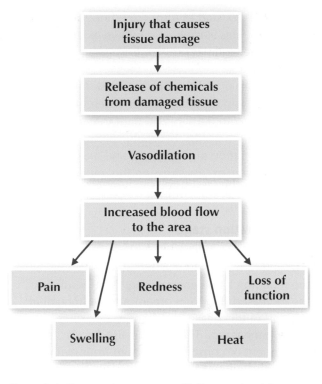

Figure 2.4: Signs and symptoms of inflammation. Why does the body react to injury in this way?

inflammation will be. This stage is also known as the acute stage.

Your main role as the sports therapist in this stage is to control the inflammation. Increased vascular activity over a prolonged period of time slows the rate of repair and can increase the risk of secondary **hypoxic** death of previously undamaged tissue (Brukner and Khan, 2006), so sustained inflammation does not aid effective recovery. During this stage you will be expected to give immediate treatment and advice.

The proliferative stage

This stage lasts for two to five weeks and is the phase of healing where new tissue is laid down at the site of injury. This early repair work is characterised by a new network of capillaries and **lymphatics** being developed, which means that the injury site now has improved circulation and drainage. After this, there is a rapid production of **fibroblasts** at the injury site which develop in the connective tissues, and are responsible for repair. Fibroblasts are the precursors to collagen, elastic fibres and reticular fibres and over the coming weeks the new tissue increases in strength as the

---

 Key terms

Vasodilation – an increase in the diameter of blood vessels that results in an increased blood flow

Hypoxia – reduced pressure of inspired oxygen, thus reducing the amount of oxygen being sent to the tissues

Lymphatic system – a network of vessels that carries lymph

Lymph – a fluid that carries water, electrolytes and proteins from the tissues

Fibroblasts – a cell in connective tissue

collagen fibres start to form cross links between each other. This stage is also known as the early repair stage, cellular proliferation stage or the sub-acute stage.

Your main role as the sports therapist during this stage is to help develop mobility exercises with your client within a safe and pain-free range. As the injury is still in a stage of repair, carefully monitor the rehabilitation of your client and make sure that you avoid any excess stress on the injured tissue as this could lead to re-injury (see *Chapter 5: Sports rehabilitation*).

The maturation stage

This stage can last from around three weeks up to a period of months and is the final phase where the repairing tissue gains strength as a result of the increased structural organisation (although at the start of this phase, the organisation of tissue is rather haphazard). This stage is also known as the subsequent or consolidation stage. Your main role as the sports therapist through this stage is to increase the level of rehabilitation, including more mobility, strengthening, flexibility, power and **proprioception** work which are all essential for the long-term functional rehabilitation of repairing tissue (see *Chapter 5: Sports rehabilitation*).

Key terms

Proprioception – the body's ability to sense movements within joints and joint positions

Progress – an injury getting better

Regress – an injury getting worse

Key principles of sports injury assessment

Injury evaluation is the first stage of treating the injury. As a sports therapist make sure that you know what you are working with before you attempt to advise, treat or rehabilitate your client. When assessing clients you will go through two processes: subjective assessment and objective assessment.

Subjective assessment

Subjective assessment of your client is the 'history taking' stage of the assessment where the client describes their injury. It is always the first stage of any client evaluation and precedes any objective

testing. However, you must try to get your client to be as clear as possible with the information that they give. This is called the subjective stage because the client is offering you information about the injury – such as how the injury has **progressed** or **regressed** since it first occurred or how much pain they have been in – you cannot be certain of the accuracy of this information as people might over-exaggerate or play down the significance of an injury.

Ask your client to elaborate on any points raised through the subjective assessment that you consider to be important for the treatment and management of the injury.

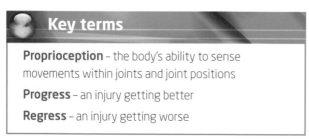

Figure 2.5: Client consultation form

Below are some suggestions for questions to ask when conducting a subjective assessment of your client, although the questions will be determined by your client's activities.

- How and when did the injury happen?
- Onset of injury. Was it sudden? Trauma?
- What were the surface/ground conditions like?
- Current signs and symptoms?

- What problems does the injury currently cause you? Are they performance related? Do they affect everyday life?
- Does anything make the symptoms better/worse?
- Do you have any pain/discomfort? If yes, locality? Type of pain? Local/referred? Constant/intermittent? What has happened with pain over last 24 hours?
- Are you taking any medication?
- General health? Recent weight loss/gains and reasons? Previous conditions? Previous injury?
- Red, yellow, blue, black, orange flags/precautions.

Objective assessment

The objective assessment is where you collect information about the injury by looking at the injury site, **palpation**, observing specific functional movements and completing any specific tests. Your aim during this stage of assessment is to determine the degree of functional losses and gains during the injury period. For more information on joint specific objective assessment, see Brukner and Khan (2006).

Observation

You will gain a better picture of the injury status if you can observe the client (and particularly the affected part) performing different types of movements. This allows you to assess progression/regression in the injury. Consider the following aspects where possible and appropriate:
- watch the player walk into your clinic or off the field – is there a limp?
- functional ability sitting/standing
- undressing/redressing items of clothing specific to the injury site.

Whether your client is standing, seated or lying, always look for and assess:
- muscle wastage
- swelling and the degree of swelling
- any previous scars
- any general lumps, cysts, bursae
- discoloration
- postural considerations (see *Chapter 5: Sports rehabilitation*)
- position of the patella
- foot position (flat, pronated, supinated?).

Palpation

Palpation is a key part of the objective assessment. When you examine your client using palpation they could be standing, sitting or lying (**prone** and **supine**). This part of the consultation has two parts: a general assessment of the tissues within the area and precise palpation to try to find areas of tension, sensitivity or any trigger points. When palpating your client you should include the following.

- Feel for heat using the back of your hand.
- Any swelling? Is it soft/hard?
- Pain? Degree of pain using pain scale (1–10). Area of pain? Type of pain?
- Palpate all bony points, ligaments, tendons, muscles, along joint lines.

Key terms

Palpation – physical assessment of tissues using precise touching and feeling

Prone – laying face down

Supine – laying down facing up

Remember

For lower limb injuries, always view the injury with the client standing if possible as this ensures weight bearing through limbs, and make sure that you view from anterior, posterior and lateral perspectives.

Always compare both sides of the body so that you can check for differences.

Movements

The final important part of your objective assessment is the movements that your client can perform. Three types of movement are used to assess the injury status: active, passive and resisted.

- Active movements are movements performed by the client.
- Passive movements are movements performed by the sports therapist (e.g. manually flexing the leg of the client at the knee).
- Resisted movements are movements performed by the client and resisted by the sports therapist.

When using these different types of movement with your client, your client should be tested through a 'pain free' movement. Consider some of these questions when working with your client:

- What range of movement is achieved pain free?
- What is the limiting factor in preventing movement?
- How does the movement gained compare to the uninjured side?

Specific testing

As part of your injury evaluation, you will need to conduct different tests to give you a better idea of the progression or regression of the injury. The tests used by sports therapists to assess injury status include range of movement testing, gait analysis, manual muscle tests and ligament stress tests.

Range of movement testing

Range of movement testing is an important part of the objective assessment as marked restrictions in movement should encourage the sports therapist to examine the injury condition further and consider possible causes (e.g. pain, swelling, muscle spasm).

Range of movement testing can be active or passive. In active range of movement testing ask your client to perform active range of movement exercises that allow you to look for restrictions in movement, the point of onset of pain or any abnormal movement patterns. Passive range of movement testing is used to bring out joint or muscle stiffness. This can be important for identifying injuries as the injury may be the cause of stiffness, or the stiffness may result in the injury. Range of movement testing should include all directions that are appropriate to a particular joint and slight over-pressure can be used at the end of the range of movement if you need to elicit your client's symptoms.

When conducting range of movement testing, compare your client's range of movement to the established norms (allowing a few degrees either side). Table 2.5 shows range of movement for different joints. Range of movement is often tested using a **goniometer**, although experienced sports therapists are often able to assess range of movement simply with a keen eye.

Key term

Goniometer – a device used to measure different joint angles

Table 2.5: Norms for range of movement at different joints

Joint	Range of Movement
Cervical	Flexion 45° Hyperextension 45° Rotation 75° Lateral flexion 50°
Shoulder	Flexion 170° Hyperextension 50° Abduction 175° Adduction 180° Medial rotation 75° Lateral rotation 90° Horizontal abduction 30° Horizontal adduction 120°
Elbow	Flexion 145° Extension 145 – 0°
Radio – Ulnar	Pronation 90° Supination 85°
Wrist	Flexion 85° Hyperextension 75° Radial deviation 25° Ulnar deviation 30°
Hip	Flexion 125° Hyperextension 20° Abduction 45° Adduction 25° Medial rotation 45° Lateral rotation 45°
Knee	Flexion 130° Extension 130 – 0°
Ankle	Dorsiflexion 20° Plantarflexion 45°
Foot	Inversion 30° Eversion 25°

Gait analysis

Gait analysis is a worthwhile procedure as an abnormal gait is usually a risk factor in injury or as a result of injury. Gait analysis is conducted most simply by observing or recording your client from anterior, posterior and lateral viewpoints so that gait patterns can be observed. In more sophisticated clinical settings, gait can be analysed using force plates that will provide ground reaction forces at different points of the gait. When conducting gait analysis with your client, they should be wearing shorts and should be measured barefoot and in trainers. If your client uses **orthotics** they should be observed walking with and without the orthotics.

As well as watching your client walk as part of the gait analysis examine the feet for pressure signs such as calluses, corns and blisters. Examine footwear for signs of uneven wear and suitability to the activity and examine feet for any signs of biomechanical abnormalities such as **pes planus**, **pes cavus**, **hallux valgus**, **varus** or **valgus** heels.

Key terms

Orthotics – corrective insoles that can either be purchased over the counter or made by prescription, used to correct gait problems Pes planus – flat foot

Pes planus – being flat footed with no noticable arch

Pes cavus – having a high foot arch

Hallux valgus – bunions

Varus – the position in which a body segment is bowed medially

Valgus – the position in which a body segment is bowed laterally

In most clients, painful gait is easy to identify as the client will have a pronounced limp, with the client taking their weight off the affected limb as quickly as possible or making a shorter stride on the affected limb. If a client has a stiff leg gait, they may abduct the leg at the hip when walking.

Manual muscle tests

These tests examine the strength of the affected and unaffected muscles and muscle groups. In manual muscle tests the client often performs isometric muscle actions against the sports therapist's resistance and the muscle is usually tested at the mid-point of movement, although isotonic muscle actions can also be tested if you wish to examine the client's functional test. The muscle contractions are normally held for approximately five seconds and repeated a few times so that the sports therapist can assess the level of weakening. This is an important element of the objective assessment as muscle weakness often accompanies injury in a given area (Hough, Lieu and Caldwell, 2011).

When conducting manual muscle testing look at the strength of contraction using a simple scale:

0 – no contraction
1 – slight contraction – trace
2 – weak contraction – poor
3 – weak contraction – fair
4 – normal contraction – good
5 – strong contraction – very good

As well as assessing the degree of strength, record if and where the client reports any pain. Observe and palpate the muscle at the same time as it is being tested.

Ligament stress test

Ligaments should be assessed for laxity and pain as part of the objective assessment. Ligament stress tests are tests that place a longitudinal stress along the length of the ligament and are often combined with palpation of the area, particularly around the insertion sites of the affected ligaments. There are a number of specific tests that have been devised for all of the major ligaments, such as the **Lachman's test** and **Anterior Drawer** test which have been identified to asses the condition of the anterior cruciate ligament (Day, Fox and Paul-Taylor, 2009). Usually, ligament laxity is graded as +1 (mild), +2 (moderate) and +3 (severe) (Bloomfield, Fricker and Fitch, 1995).

Remember

Always tell your client what you are doing and why you are doing it – communication is essential to make your client feel at ease.

Key terms

Lachman's test – a test performed with the knee in 15° flexion where the examiner draws the tibia forward, assessing the joint for laxity

Anterior drawer test – a test performed with the knee in 90° flexion and the client's foot kept stable. The tibia is drawn forward and the joint is assessed for degree of movement and quality of end point

Activity

You are working with an athletics club which has had a number of injuries among their youth athletes. The athletes that have been injured are mainly representing the club in either 100 m sprint, triple jump, discus and 10,000 m. As a result of this, you have decided to investigate the sports further so that you can get a greater understanding of the different impacts of the sports on injury occurrence. In order to do this, answer the following questions.

1 What are the physical, physiological and psychological demands of each of the different events?

2 What are the likely causes of injury that are associated with each of the different events?

3 What are the different types of injury that are likely to occur in the different events?

4 What are the key preventative measures that can be put in place for these different events?

Case study

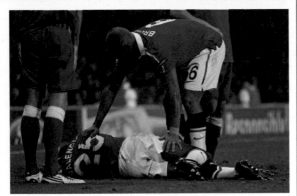

A serious injury that is often suffered by footballers and rugby players is a twist (sprain) of the ankle or knee. This type of ankle injury can be relatively minor or can lead to other tissues becoming damaged, such as fracture or dislocation in the most severe cases.

This type of injury was suffered by England Rugby international Danny Cipriani in 2008, Croatian footballer Eduardo, in 2008 and England footballer Alan Smith in 2006.

Questions

1. What do you think are the mechanisms of this type of injury?

2. What will be the signs and symptoms of injury?

3. What will be the body's response to injury?

4. What preventative measures (if any) could be put in place?

5. How would you tackle assessing such a serious and sensitive injury?

6. What are your limitations of practice in this case?

Check your understanding

1. Give a definition of sports injury.

2. Why might soccer have the highest rate of injury across the world?

3. How would you classify a hamstring strain caused by sudden acceleration in 100 m sprinting?

4. What is the difference between an intrinsic and extrinsic risk factor?

5. List five extrinsic risk factors of injury associated with cricket.

6. What is the difference between an overuse injury and an acute injury?

7. How can regular fitness testing prevent sports injuries?

8. Name three common injuries a rugby union player could sustain.

9. What are the key stages of the inflammatory process?

10. Why would you use subjective and objective assessment together?

To obtain answers to these questions visit the companion website at www.pearsonfe.co.uk/foundationsinsport

Useful resources

To obtain a secure link to the websites below, see the Websites section on page ii or visit the companion website at www.pearsonfe.co.uk/foundationsinsport.

British Journal of Sports Medicine
Virtual Sports Injury Clinic
Sports Injury Bulletin
SportEx Medicine

Further reading

Anderson, M.K., Hall, S.J., & Parr, G.P. (2008) *Foundations of Athletic Training: Prevention, Assessment, and Management*. 4th Ed. Philadelphia: Lippincott, Williams & Wilkins.

Baher, R. & Holme, I. (2003). Risk Factors for Sports Injuries: A Methodological Approach. *British Journal of Sports Medicine,* Vol. 37, 384–392.

Bahr, R. & Maehlum, L. (2004) *Clinical Guide to Sports Injuries*. Champaign: Human Kinetics.

Bloomfield, J., Fricker, P.A., and Fitch, K.D. (1995). *Science and Medicine in Sport*. London: Blackwell Science.

Bronner, S., Ojofeitimi, S., and Mayers, L. (2006). Comprehensive Surveillance of Dance Injuries. *Journal of Dance, Medicine and Science*, Vol. 10, 69–80.

Brukner, P. & Khan, K. (2006) *Clinical Sports Medicine,* 3rd Ed. Sydney: McGraw-Hill.

Cartwright, L.A. & Pitney, W.A. (2005) *Fundamentals of Athletic Training*: 2nd Ed. Champaign: Human Kinetics.

Day, R., Fox, J., and Paul-Taylor, G. (2009). *Neuro-Musculoskeletal Clinical Tests: A Clinician's Guide*. London: Churchill Livingstone.

Emery, C.A., Rose, M.S., McAllister, J.R., and Meeuwisse, W.H. (2007). A Prevention Strategy to Reduce the Incidence of Injury in High-School Basketball. *Clinical Journal of Sports Medicine*, Vol. 17, 17–24.

Fredericson, M., and Wolf, C. (2005). Iliotibialband Syndrome in Runners: Innovation in Treatment. *Sports Medicine*, Vol. 35, 451–459.

Goggs, R., et al. (2005). Neutraceutical Therapies for Degenerative Joint Diseases: A Critical Review. *Critical Reviews in Food Science and Nutrition*, Vol. 45, 145–164.

Gross, J.M., Fetto, J., & Rosen, E. (2002) *Musculoskeletal Examination* 2nd Ed. Oxford: Blackwell Science.

Hough, C.L., Lieu, B.K., and Caldwell, E.S. (2011). Manual Muscle Strength Testing of Critically Ill Patients: Feasibility and Interobserver Agreement. *Critical Care*, Vol. 15, 1–18.

Kolt, G.S., & Snyder-Mackler, L. (2005*) Physical Therapies in Sport and Exercise*. 2nd Ed. Elsevier Limited.

Kroll, T., Neri, M.T., and Ho, P-S. (2007). Secondary Conditions in Spinal Cord Injury: Results from a Prospective Study. *Disability and Rehabilitation*, Vol. 29, 1229–1237.

Lewis, G., Schwellnus, M.P., and Sole, G. (2000). The Etiology and Clinical Features of Lower Back Pain in Distance Runners: A Review. *International SportMed Journal*, Vo. 4, 1–25.

Norris, C. (2004) *Sports Injuries: Diagnosis and Management*: 3rd Ed. London: Butterworth and Heinemann.

Shamus, E. & Shamus, J. (2001) *Sports Injury: Prevention and Rehabilitation*. Philadelphia: Lippincott, Williams & Wilkins.

Shultz, S.J., Houglum, P.A., and Perrin, D.H., (2005) *Examination of Musculoskeletal Injuries* 2nd Ed. Champaign: Human Kinetics.

Starkey, C. (2000). Injuries and Illness in the National Basketball Association. *Journal of Athletic Training*, Vol. 35, 161–167.

Walker, B. (2007) *The Anatomy of Sports Injuries*. Chichester: Lotus Publishing.

Ward, K. (2004) *Hands on Sports Therapy*. London: Thomson Learning.

Whyte, G. (2006). *The Physiology of Training*. London: Churchill Livingstone Elsevier.

Chapter 3

Fundamentals of sports massage

Introduction

Any regular participation in sport and exercise has major effects on the soft tissues and connective tissues of the body. Not all these effects are desirable and they can have a profound effect on an athlete's performance, their chances of getting injured and quality of daily living. Negative effects include:

- muscle soreness and prolonged elevation of muscle tightness
- micro trauma to soft tissue
- muscle imbalance and asymmetry
- reduced flexibility and range of movement (ROM)
- feelings of lethargy and exhaustion.

As a result of these, there is a need for a treatment or intervention to help athletes to train and compete at their best, and maintain a good quality of life. Sports massage is a relatively new discipline, although the use of massage in sport dates back to the ancient Olympics. Sports massage is a type of manual soft tissue therapy that is applied in a sport and exercise context and which is gaining popularity across many sports. Professional bodies in sports therapy view it as an essential skill in the prehabilitation of athletes and the treatment, and rehabilitation of athletes suffering from sports injury.

Learning outcomes

After you have read this chapter you should be able to:

- describe the aims of sports massage
- explain the major benefits of sports massage
- describe contraindications to sports massage
- describe how to prepare for sports massage
- explain the stages of a client consultation
- explain how to conduct sports massage techniques
- describe the benefits of sports massage techniques
- explain the principles of pre- and post-event massage.

It is not unusual for athletes at any level to train and/or compete most days of the week. This repetitive overloading of the body has many physiological and psychological effects.

- List the various physiological and psychological effects of regular sport and exercise participation.

- List how regular sports massage might have a benefit on these effects.

- What are the knowledge requirements of a sports massage therapist?

The aims of sports massage

Sports massage is a flexible way of treating athletes and other clients. It can be delivered in a variety of environments and conducted before, during and after training and competition to aid performance and promote recovery in an athlete's rehabilitation programme. Ultimately, sports massage is conducted to achieve one or more of the following aims, i.e. to:

- prevent sport- and exercise-related injury
- improve performance in training and competition
- improve recovery from training and competition
- improve recovery and rehabilitation from sport- and exercise-related injury
- maintain an athlete's well-being.

The major benefits of sports massage

The popularity of sports massage within the athletic world for performance and health benefits is growing. There is a lack of strong statistical data, but there is strong subjective evidence including testimonies from athletes and other sports professionals that suggests sports massage is a valuable and effective form of treatment. The major focus of sports massage is to manipulate **soft tissues**. However, as a treatment, sports massage affects a number of interlinking physiological systems such as:

- the muscular system
- the skeletal system
- the cardiovascular system
- the nervous system
- the lymphatic system
- the digestive and urinary system.

As sports massage affects most of the essential physiological systems of the body, it can have a wide variety of benefits. These not only aid athletic life but can improve the quality of normal everyday living and health. For example, sports massage may reduce the effect of muscle soreness post competition and allow for less interruption to training for an athlete; in the general population, it can reduce the effect of lower back pain for manual workers and prevent other chronic conditions such as osteoarthritis and postural problems.

Each sports massage technique has its own proposed purpose and benefit. Most of the benefits of sports massage to athletes are anecdotal and lack a strong evidence base. The widely believed general benefits of sports massage can be broadly categorised as:

- mechanical
- physiological
- psychological (Brukner and Khan, 2006).

Mechanical benefits – It is thought that sports massage may enhance the way the body moves. By improving mobility and range of movement an athlete will be able to execute techniques more effectively and safely. Swelling, **adhesions**, and the general tension associated with training and competition can reduce an athlete's mobility. Sports massage can help mobilise more muscle fibres so athletic movements can be performed with more speed and power (Brukner and Khan, 2006). The process of being touched and recognising pain, tightness and tension could also give an athlete more **kinaesthetic awareness**.

Soft tissues – a general term to describe tissues of the muscles, ligaments, and tendons

Adhesions – bands of fibrous tissue formed between muscle fibres

Kinaesthetic awareness – a sensory skill that your body uses to know where it is in open space

Physiological benefits – sports massage may have a profound effect on the major physiological systems of the body (Findlay, 2010). By stimulating these systems above resting levels, and improving local area metabolism, sports massage can help to improve sports performance, recovery from training and competing, and rehabilitation from injury (Stasinopoulos and Johnson, 2004). For example, increasing blood flow to an injured area is thought to decrease recovery time, and increasing **lymph flow** is thought to reduce the time in the inflammatory stage of healing. In many ways, conducting a sports massage can have a similar effect to a warm-up and cool-down in terms of increasing blood flow and facilitating the removal of waste products (Monedero and Donne, 2000; Jakeman, Byrne, and Eston, 2010).

Psychological benefits – sports massage may enhance cognition, emotion, and behaviour of the athlete. It can help with the mood disturbances and feelings of exhaustion that accompany regular participation (Ernst, 1998; Hemmings, Smith, Graydon, and Dyson, 2000). Massage can relax or stimulate depending on an athlete's individual needs. Before competition an athlete may need a vigorous massage to stimulate or alternatively an anxious athlete may require a massage to relax them in order to help them to perform well. Perception of injury-induced pain may be reduced by the increase in temperature caused by improvements in local area blood flow. Sports massage may improve self confidence by giving an athlete a feeling of ease with sporting movement with less risk of injury. Whether or not the psychological benefit of sports massage is merely a **placebo effect** needs to be further researched.

Table 3.1: A summary of the proposed benefits of sports massage

Mechanical	Physiological	Psychological
• Loosens adhesions • Reduces tension • Reduces oedema • Improves posture • Increases flexibility • Stretches soft tissue • Reduces stress on joints • Mobilisation of muscle fibres • Improved kinaesthetic awareness	• Increases lymph flow • Improves local area blood flow • Removes waste products • Promotes healing • Increases parasympathetic activity • Pain reduction relating to hormones	• Reduces anxiety • Reduces tension • Relaxing/ stimulating • Reduces pain • Elevates mood • Gives better attentional focus • Improves sleep • Improves confidence

(Brukner and Khan, 2006 and Findlay, 2010)

Contraindications to sports massage

There may be situations where sports massage is contraindicated and can be ill-advised with certain clients. The word **contraindication** in a sports massage setting means conditions which mean you cannot continue with the treatment, or need to modify the treatment plan. Not all contraindications are absolute, i.e. they do not always mean that a sports massage cannot be delivered. For example, if a client has a verruca it does not mean sports massage cannot be conducted but that the treatment may be modified in some way. It is not uncommon for a client to present more than one contraindication. For example, an athlete who has diabetes may also have fungal infections of the feet. A sports therapist must know exactly:

- when to refer a client to another professional
- when a sports massage is ill-advised
- when and how a treatment needs to be modified.

For more detail on the pathology of sports massage contraindications see Werner (2009).

Key terms

Lymph flow – the rate of supply and removal of lymph fluid

Placebo effect – a treatment which has no objective benefit but which produces a subjective perception of a therapeutic effect

Contraindication – a condition or factor that speaks against a certain measure, medication or treatment

When providing sports massage in any setting the following contraindications must be understood:

- red flag
- global
- local
- modifying.

Red flag contraindications

Red flag contraindications mean that a sports massage must not be conducted and the client must be referred to an appropriate healthcare professional (usually a GP) immediately. Once the healthcare professional has medically assessed the client, and formally stated that a sports massage can be conducted, then you can proceed with caution. Red flag contraindications include the following:

- Undiagnosed conditions – a client may disclose that they have an undiagnosed condition or present common symptoms of one. The condition could be made worse by sports massage and is completely beyond limitations of practice. An injury with symptoms of loss of sensation or abnormal bodily function can mean blood flow or nervous interruption and should always be referred as a precaution. For example, a client presenting symptoms of breathlessness, fatigue, swelling of the hands and feet, poor sleep and sharp pain in the limbs, may have an undiagnosed heart or circulatory condition and must be referred immediately to a GP. The same principle applies for undiagnosed lumps, suspicious looking moles, and suspected **thrombosis**.

- Unstable conditions – those that are not predictable and not controlled. This means that the aggravating factors have not been established, and medication is not yet effective. A sports massage may aggravate the symptoms of this condition and place a client in danger. Common examples include uncontrolled **hypertension** or angina.

- Changes in sensation – for example, acute headache (with no obvious cause), numbness, pins and needles, palpitations and sudden dizziness. These can indicate that a client may have an underlying cardiovascular or neural issue that requires medical treatment. If these symptoms are present after trauma such as a sports injury or a car crash the client must be referred immediately.

- Changes in function – these include slurred speech, drop attacks, disturbed sleep and changes in bowel or urinary function. They could point to an underlying cardiovascular or neural issue and the client must be referred, especially if post-trauma.

Key terms

Thrombosis – the formation of a blood clot inside a blood vessel, obstructing the flow of blood through the circulatory system

Hypertension – a chronic medical condition in which the systemic arterial blood pressure is elevated

Top tip

Although there is a certain amount of clinical judgement needed with red flag contraindications it is far better to be cautious and refer on to protect yourself and the client.

Global contraindications

Global contraindications prevent a sports massage until a healthcare professional formally states otherwise. These conditions tend to be complex, high risk, severe, contagious and acute. Clients with these conditions may be on strong medication which might have contraindications to sports massage. The type and dosage of medication must be checked in the British National Formulatory (BNF) or if unsure the client should be referred.

See Table 3.2 for a list of conditions that carry global contraindications.

Local contraindications

These conditions do not necessarily rule out a sports massage but you should proceed with great caution. Particular care is needed when you are considering the area to be massaged, the positioning of the client, the techniques to be used and the massage medium. With a number of these conditions you need to ensure that the application of sports massage is not detrimental to the healing process.

Conditions that can be classified as local contraindications are shown in Table 3.2.

Modifying contraindications

A sports massage can be conducted but the treatment must be modified to compensate for these conditions. Sports massage is largely beneficial for these conditions. However, care must be taken so that neither you nor the client are at risk. Risks to the sports therapist would be associated with infectious disease and litigation if an incorrect or inappropriate treatment was carried out. Risks to the client would be that the treatment given may bring on adverse symptoms of their condition. Clear modifications that need to be addressed with these conditions are client positioning, choice of techniques, depth of massage, direction and intensity of massage, duration of massage, stage of tissue healing and massage medium used.

Conditions that can be classified as those requiring modification of the treatment are shown opposite in Table 3.2.

> ### Top tip
>
> A thorough client assessment is needed to ensure a client reveals all contraindications to sports massage so a safe and effective treatment plan can be formulated.

Table 3.2: Global, local and modifying contraindications

Global	Local	Modifying
• Strong medications (side effects) • Peripheral vascular disease • Compartment syndrome • Contagious disease (e.g. flu, cold) • Haemophilia • Shock • Phlebitis • Under the influence of alcohol or recreational drugs • Acute injuries (allow 72 hours) • Severe pain • Cardiovascular disease • Acute angina • Tumours • Recent major surgery • Impetigo	• Haematoma (inter and intra muscular • Fractures • Varicose veins • Metal pins and plates • Fungal infections • Contusions • Dermatitis • Acne • Eczema • Sunburn • Verrucas • Myositis ossificans • Open wounds • Melanoma	• Pregnancy • Minor recent surgery • Asthma • HIV/AIDS • Diabetes (type 1 and 2) • Allergies • Arthritis (osteo and rheumatoid) • Cancer • Multiple sclerosis • Cystic fibrosis • Osteoporosis

(Findlay, 2010)

Preparing for sports massage

Proper preparation prevents poor professional performance. This well-known phrase also applies to carrying out sports massage. Careful preparation means that a sports massage can be effectively conducted and that you and the client are not put at risk (for example, from faulty equipment or cross-infection). Preparing for a sports massage involves:

- the practitioner and equipment
- the environment/venue
- the client or athletes

The practitioner and equipment

Good hygiene standards are essential for any healthcare profession. Professional bodies such as the Society of Sports Therapists include the need to establish and maintain a safe working environment in their benchmark standards of proficiency. The challenge for sports massage is the maintenance of good hygiene standards across all the environments where it is conducted. For example, there are differences in how hygiene is addressed in a clinic setting (where everything can be controlled) compared to on the field of play during an event or in a changing room before an event. You should be extremely careful not to transmit an infection to your client and vice versa. Broadly, infection can be transmitted:

- indirectly through equipment, coaches, regularly used surfaces
- directly through touch, handshakes, bodily fluid
- airborne (for example, the flu and cold virus).

In order to keep yourself and your environment hygienic conside the following questions.

- Are you and client in good health and free from viruses?
- Have you washed your hands correctly before and after treatment?
- Are you wearing clean attire?
- Is the equipment, e.g. couch, face hole and floor clean?
- Are clean towels and a clean couch roll being used?
- Is your massage medium fresh and new?
- Are your nails short and have you removed jewellery that can harbour bacteria?
- Has bodily fluid been disposed of correctly?
- Are common areas of contact cleaned regularly?

It is essential that you dress and present yourself as a professional. This establishes your credibility as a knowledgeable and skilled professional and puts the client at ease. Quite often clients will expect the person conducting a sports massage to be a role model and practise what they preach. How might a client react if their sports massage was being conducted by someone who smelt of cigarette smoke or alcohol?

Stop and think

Think how a sports therapist should look when conducting a sports massage and create a code of practice for personal and professional skills.

Effective sport massage often involves physically demanding movements. You need to adopt a good working posture to reduce strain on your joints, soft tissues and connective tissues. Using a good working posture uses larger muscle groups to exert force and reduces demand on smaller structures that may become damaged. If it is not maintained then any manual lifting of clients, or repetitively assuming a poor posture when massaging, could lead to problems and time off work. Good posture ensures that you are able to work effectively and for a much longer period of time.

Generally a good working posture in sports massage follows these principles.

- Generate movement using your legs, not your arms, so that your small muscle groups do not fatigue early or get damaged.
- Massage with a wide stance (feet around 90 cm apart) to give better balance and use larger muscle groups more effectively.
- Keep your shoulders and hips in line with the direction of your technique to prevent unnatural repetitive twisting movements.
- Try to ensure you do not lock out your elbows at the end of a massage stroke to reduce strain on joint components.
- Think about the shape of your back. Try to keep it as neutral as possible.
- Before you lift or manually handle a client, consider the realistic strength you need to do it. If you do decide to lift a client's limbs, push from your legs.
- If you are using a couch ensure it is at the correct height based on client size and the technique you are using. The couch height should generally be just below hip height.

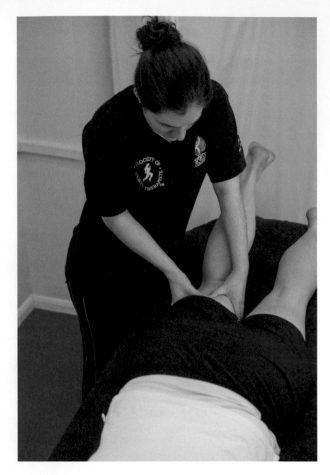

Figure 3.1: Effective working posture; conducting a sports massage on the hamstring group

The environment/venue

Ideally a sports massage venue will be comfortable, secure, safe, spacious, clean, private and well ventilated. However this is not always the case. Sports massage can be conducted at a wide range of venues and environments such as in clinics, in changing rooms, in clients' homes and on the field of play. Ensuring these venues are as safe as possible for you and the client is essential.

As sports massage has a profound effect on the physiological systems of the body, a well-kept and maintained first aid kit should be available together with nearby phone access if the emergency services are needed. All massaging venues and environments should have a risk assessment to identify risks,

hazards, and preventative measures. The working area should be free from obstacles and fire doors kept clear. You and your client should be aware of emergency procedures in case of fire or bomb danger.

The client/athlete

Preparing the client will ensure a sports massage treatment is both safe and effective for all parties involved. Clients need to be fully informed about the treatment they will undergo. Sports massage can cause discomfort both during and after treatment. You should brief a client on what sports massage can do for them and its limitations. This means that clients will not place you in an awkward position and will respect you as a professional. If working with athletes (especially children) you should convey this information to parents, carers, or coaches as well as the athletes themselves. Give your client advice that covers:

- what to wear during the massage

- the benefits and limitations of sports massage

- an understanding that, if the client's health changes in any way, they must inform you as this could affect the treatment plan.

Stages of a client consultation

An effective client consultation is necessary before a sports massage is conducted. A good consultation should provide you with enough information to safely and effectively manage a client's treatment and place the client at ease by explaining how sports massage can benefit them.

A thorough client assessment has three stages: subjective assessment, objective assessment and the reasoning/planning stage. More thorough coverage about the process of a client assessment can be seen in *Chapter 2: Introduction to sports injury and assessment*. Table 3.3 identifies the major components in each of these stages.

Table 3.3: The key components of a sports massage consultation

Subjective assessment	Objective assessment	Reasoning/planning

• Personal details
• Healthcare professional details (if referred)
• Other treatments received
• Medical background
• Medication
• Activity history
• Lifestyle history
• About the major problem:
  - when?
  - causes?
  - symptoms?
  - pain?
  - aggravating factors?
	• Pain scale and type
	• Postural analysis
	• Palpation of affected area
	• Range of movement tests and comparison
	• Muscle function tests and comparison
	• **Bilateral comparison** for symptoms
		• Contraindications?
		• Side effects of medication
		• Likely cause
		• Referral?
		• Selecting from a range of effective techniques
		• Use of all information to formulate a plan of action
		• Verbalise specific benefits of the plan to the client

When assessing or reassessing a client you should use **outcome measures**. This means that initial client limitations and progressions can be qualified and quantified. For example, an outcome measure of joint mobility is using **goniometry** to assess improvements in degrees of movement at individual joints. Evaluating a massage treatment forms part of National Occupational Standards (NOS) for Sports Massage D520 and D521. By using well-established outcome measures, the use of sports massage in both the athletic and non-athletic world will become more important.

Key terms

Bilateral comparison – the process of checking signs, symptoms and function on both the affected and non-affected side

Outcome measures – using subjective and objective measures post treatment to evaluate and measure improvements

Goniometry – the measuring of angles created by the bones of the body at the joints

Stop and think

Relating to NOS D520 and D521, how could you subjectively and objectively evaluate massage methods?

Conducting sports massage techniques

Before sports massage, a treatment plan needs to be drawn up which includes:

- client positioning
- massage medium
- massage techniques.

Top tip

Always ask the client if they have a nut allergy as certain massage mediums are made from nut oils. If in doubt use hypoallergenic forms of lubrication.

Client positioning

There are four ways in which a client can be positioned for sports massage. All of these positions should be comfortable, safe and allow good access for the practitioner. The four positions are:

- client laid in supine position on a couch, floor or on a bench
- client laid in prone position on a couch, floor or on a bench
- client laid in a side position on a couch, floor or on a bench
- client sitting up in a seated position.

- **Supine position** (client on their back) – a cushion should be placed under the head and knees for support. This allows the client to remain in a neutral position for the massage and prevent the knee joint from being **hyperextended**.

- **Prone position** (client on their front) – cushions should be placed under the ankles and under the abdominals. This will prevent the ankles from being hyperflexed and relax the gastrocnemius and hamstrings for sports massage. Placing a cushion under the abdominals will very slightly flex the spine and relax the lower back muscles. The cushion under the abdominals is especially important if the client has lower back or postural problems.

- **Side facing position** – careful consideration of the alignment of the body is needed. Ideally a cushion should be placed at the side of the head to keep the cervical vertebrae in a neutral position. The client's top leg should be placed at 90° and a cushion placed under this also. The lower leg should be straight allowing for the lower back and pelvis to be kept in alignment.

- **Seated position** – the client's feet must be able to rest flat on the floor. Ensure the client maintains a **neutral vertebrae** and to facilitate this a cushion can be used as a support. Being able to conduct a seated sports massage is useful when working with disabled clients or those that are unable to easily manoeuvre themselves onto the couch, for example pregnant women.

Key terms

Hyperextension – extending a joint beyond its normal range of movement (it is associated with injury)

Neutral vertebrae – the proper alignment of the body between postural extremes. In its natural alignment, the spine is not straight – it has natural curves in the thoracic (upper) and lumbar (lower) regions

Top tip

Too little lubrication will irritate hair follicles, while too much will reduce any friction which you are trying to gain to increase circulation.

Massage medium

Table 3.4: The range of possible massage mediums and basic implications of use

Massage medium	Implications
Oil	Provides long-lasting lubrication Can be infused with relaxing/stimulating additives Be aware of oils made from nuts because of client allergies
Cream	Use on hirsute clients to prevent folliculitis (irritated hair follicles) Usually requires a number of applications Tends to be more hypoallergenic
Talcum powder	Good for pre-event massage Provides greater friction Messy to use

Massage techniques

Palpation

This helps to locate areas of pain, adhesions and muscle spasm. The thumb is used to differentiate between soft tissues that are in a normal healthy condition and those that have been placed under excessive strain or damaged in some way. Initially you may observe a particular problem area for the client and use palpation to prove or disprove your thoughts.

Effleurage

This is the technique that begins a treatment and is returned to throughout. It can be delivered superficially at the start or deeply throughout the treatment. Usually it is used to quickly warm the muscle tissue and spread the lubricant. Using the palmer surface (palms) of the hands with passive thumbs direct pressure should be applied from **distal** to **proximal** (or in the general direction of the heart) followed by a significantly lighter returning stroke. When using effleurage care should be taken when massaging over joints with a reduction of pressure needed so that structures such as blood vessels and lymph glands are not damaged.

Key terms

Distal – further away from the centre of the body

Proximal – towards the centre of the body

Petrissage

This includes a range of kneading type techniques aimed at lifting, pressing, and releasing muscle tissue. Like effleurage this can be applied superficially or more deeply. It is generally used after effleurage to further warm the muscle tissues by applying deeper pressure. Again in these techniques the thumbs should be passive (saving them for more specific areas). Classic petrissage techniques are:

- circular petrissage – create a circular position with hands and arms with elbows out – conduct a continuous circular pressurised movement

- wringing petrissage – the pressure from one hand moving towards the muscles midline is matched by the other hand moving in the opposite direction

- kneading petrissage – this consists of manipulating the muscle tissues in a circular manner, involving lifting and squeezing the muscles. As one hand releases its grip the other hand takes up a grip adjacent to it.

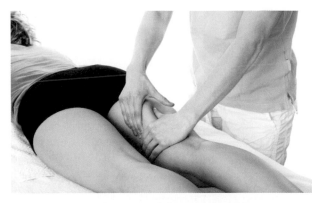

Figure 3.2: An example of wringing petrissage to the hamstring group

Remember

All sports massage techniques can be applied more vigorously and deeply depending on the client's needs and stage of the treatment.

Compression

This is a flexible technique that can be used in normal sports massage or through clothes. Its aim is to compress the muscle tissue to increase blood flow and warm it up through compression and relaxation. Compressions should be conducted at 45° so that the muscle is not pressed onto the bone. The movement using the palm of the hands, thumbs or fist (depending on the depth required and muscle) involves pushing down on the muscle tissues followed by a slow release.

Frictions

These are used to break down adhesions and scar tissue leading to healthy aligned muscle fibres and can also facilitate recovery from injury. Frictions can cause more discomfort than any of the techniques outlined above – so regular communication is vital with the client. (For example, you could use a pain scale of 1–10.) Frictions can be circular if you are using them on muscle and transverse if you are using them on tendon or ligament. Frictions are normally conducted using the thumbs or reinforced index finger. Simply apply gentle direct pressure to the affected area producing very small and slow movements (maintaining the original pressure). Gradually increase the pressure of the frictions every few minutes until you are affecting deep tissue. Frictions can be applied for up to 20 minutes on an affected area. Care must be taken not to overwork the area as it is easy to damage the client's tissues.

Tapotement

This is another flexible technique that can be used in a normal sports massage treatment or dry over clothes. It aims to increase local area blood flow and stimulate nerve endings. Tapotement includes a number of separate techniques that are rhythmical and require co-ordinating movements with the hands. The speed of these techniques can be altered depending on the intended outcome of the treatment. These techniques include:

- hacking – involves using the medial border of each hand with the fingers and wrists loose (not rigid). In a rhythmical fashion each hand and finger hits the muscle tissue continuously one after the other

- cupping – involves making a cup shape with the palms of the hands. Place them so the palm of the hand faces the client's muscles. Then rhythmically strike the tissue continuously, one hand after the other. This technique produces a hollow, not slapping, sound

- beating – involves making a loose fist with thumbs resting (passive) at the side of the fist shape. With the palms of the hands facing down, or fists in a vertical position, the muscle is hit in a rhythmical manner. This is usually used on larger muscle groups only.

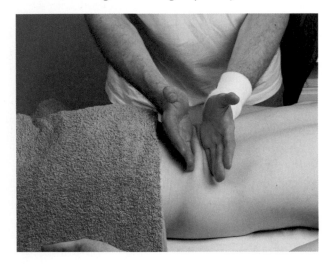

Figure 3.3: An example of hacking to the lower back

Remember

In addition to using the palm surface of the hands, additional pressure can be applied by using reinforced hands, thumbs, or bony ulna border, heel of the hand and elbow.

The benefits of sports massage techniques

You need to be able to explain why each massage technique is being used. Table 3.5 summarises the major benefits.

Table 3.5: The proposed benefit and purpose of different sports massage techniques

Sports massage technique	Proposed benefit/effect
Superficial effleurage	Warms muscles by increasing local area blood flow Disperses massage medium Stimulates lymph flow and lymph drainage Stimulates nerve endings Psychologically relaxing Pain relief
Deep effleurage	Increased removal of waste products Increased local area blood and lymph flow Increased venous return Greater relaxation of tense muscle tissue Can begin to stretch muscle fibres
Petrissage	Reduction in muscle tension Increased blood and lymph flow Separates tissues, e.g. scar tissue, fascia, adhesions Pain relief Can begin to stretch muscle fibres
Compressions	Increase in local area blood and lymph flow Greater waste product removal Decreases muscle tension and spasm Pain relief
Frictions	Decreases muscle tension and spasm Realigns fibres thus restores muscle function Breaks down adhesions and scar tissue Increases local area blood flow Can desensitise pain receptors Improves kinaesthetic awareness
Tapotement	Stimulates nerve endings (sensory receptors) Stimulates the client Increased local area blood flow Stimulates muscle contraction Improves kinaesthetic awareness

(Findlay, 2010)

Principles of pre- and post-event massage

Of particular interest to athletes is how sports massage can be used before an event to prepare for activity, during an event to maintain performance and after an event to aid recovery.

Stop and think

There is a belief that sports massage could be used as an alternative to a traditional athletic warm-up. Compare the general physiological and psychological effects of sports massage and a traditional warm-up.

Pre-event

A pre-event massage will prepare an athlete both physiologically and psychologically for activity. It can be conducted anything from a few days to a few minutes before activity. Pre-event massage aims to:

- warm up and increase local area circulation in specific muscles
- decrease muscle tension
- increase range of movement and joint mobility
- increase neural stimulation to specific muscles, giving a state of readiness
- reduce anxiety and stimulate.

Generally a pre-event massage is performed within a few hours of activity and lasts for 10–15 minutes. Techniques suitable for pre-event massage include effleurage, petrissage, compression and tapotement. The techniques can be performed quickly to stimulate an athlete or slowly to calm the athlete down if they are over anxious.

Stop and think

Which techniques would you never use in a post-event massage and why?

Table 3.6: An example of a 10–15 minute pre-event massage of the leg muscles

Legs (anterior)	Legs (posterior)
• Effleurage to whole leg (ankle to hip) • Effleurage to thigh • Petrissage to thigh • Petrissage to adductors • Effleurage to upper thigh • Tapotement to thigh and adductors • Effleurage to lower leg • Stretching of hamstrings and calf muscles (8 seconds maximum)	• Effleurage to whole leg (heel to buttocks) • Effleurage to hamstrings • Petrissage to hamstrings • Tapotement to hamstrings • Effleurage to whole leg • Effleurage to calf area (gastrocnemius, soleus, Achilles tendon) • Petrissage to calf area • Effleurage to calf area • Tapotement to calf area • Stretching of quadriceps (8 seconds maximum)

Post-event

The most common form of event massage is post event. It is thought to be important in aiding recovery from training and competition. Post-event massage aims to:

- remove waste products from specific muscles
- prevent muscle soreness
- normalise the muscle tissue
- support metabolic recovery and lymph flow
- restore flexibility and joint mobility
- check for post-event tissue damage.

A post-event massage should take place within two hours of activity and last for approximately 15–20 minutes. Techniques used in a post-event massage are: effleurage, petrissage and gentle compression, followed by active or passive stretching (lasting for 20–30 seconds). The techniques are performed much more slowly than in pre-event to help restore the body to resting conditions. The stretching is vital in restoring or improving flexibility and joint movement.

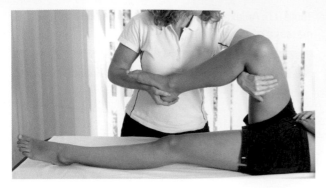

Figure 3.4: An example of passive stretching a client's hamstring muscles post-event

Table 3.7: An example of a 15–20 minute post-event massage of the leg muscles (note that techniques are applied slowly)

Legs (anterior)	Legs (posterior)
• Effleurage to whole leg (ankle to hip) • Effleurage to thigh • Slow petrissage to thigh • Effleurage to upper thigh • Effleurage to adductors • Slow petrissage to adductors • Effleurage to lower leg • Stretching of hamstrings and calf muscles (20–30 seconds)	• Effleurage to whole leg (heel to buttocks) • Effleurage to hamstrings • Slow petrissage to hamstrings • Effleurage to calf area • Slow petrissage to calf area • Effleurage to whole leg • Stretching of quadriceps muscles (20–30 seconds)

Case study

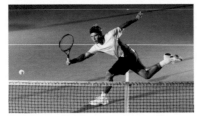

During the ATP tennis season a tennis player is consistently training, competing and travelling from one world city to the next. On occasions he arrives at a tournament only one day before the first round of an event. This tough schedule is having a profound effect on his physiology and psychology. For example, the tennis player has a long injury history and regularly feels physically and mentally exhausted. In addition he complains to the media that he is struggling to get 'psyched up' for performing and this is making him vulnerable in the opening few games and sets. You have been asked by the tennis player's coaching team to persuade him that sports massage could be beneficial.

1. Explain the specific physiological, physical and psychological benefits of sports massage to this client.

2. Which sports massage types and techniques would you use on the tennis player and why?

3. Create and justify a massage treatment plan for the tennis player. This relates to National Occupational Standard D520: Plan, apply and evaluate massage methods.

Check your understanding

1. Define sports massage.

2. Which type of tissue does a sports massage practitioner manipulate?

3. Describe the general aims of sports massage.

4. Which three categories can the benefits of sports massage be placed into?

5. Explain why a knowledge of contraindications is vital to a sports massage practitioner.

6. Describe under which conditions a client must be referred to a medical professional.

7. Explain the three stages of an effective client consultation.

8. Explain how a sports massage practitioner can maintain good hygiene standards.

9. Describe the main reasons for performing frictions on a client.

10. Explain the major aims of pre- and post-event massage.

To obtain answers to these questions visit the companion website at www.pearsonfe.co.uk/foundationsinsport

Useful resources

To obtain a secure link to the websites below, see the Websites section on page ii or visit the companion website at www.pearsonfe.co.uk/foundationsinsport.

Sports Massage Association

Virtual Sports Injury Clinic

Sports massage information from Brian Mackenzie

Society of Sports Therapists

Further reading

Benjamin, P.J. and Lamp, S.P. (2004). *Understanding Sports Massage*. Champaign: Human Kinetics.

Brukner, P. and Khan, K. (2006). *Clinical Sports Medicine* 3rd Edition. New York: McGraw Hill.

Cash, M. (1996). *Sport and Remedial Massage Therapy*. London: Ebury Press.

Dinsdale, N. (2009). Evidence-based Massage Part 1. *sportEx Dynamics*, Vol. 22, 12–17.

Dinsdale, N. (2010). Evidence-based Massage Part 2. *sportEx Dynamics*, Vol. 23, 10–13.

Ernst, E. (1998). Does post-exercise massage treatment reduce delayed onset of muscle soreness? A systematic review. *British Journal of Sports Medicine*.Vol. 32: 212–214

Findlay, S. (2010). *Sports Massage*. Champaign: Human Kinetics.

McGillicuddy, M. (2010). *Massage for Sports Performance*. Champaign: Human Kinetics.

Hemmings, B., Smith, M., Graydon, J., and Dyson, R. (2000). Effect of massage on physiological restoration, perceived recovery, and repeated sprint performance. *British Journal of Sports Medicine*. Vol. 34: 109–114

Jakeman, J.R., Byrne, C., and Eston, R.G. (2010). Efficacy of lower limb compression and combined treatment of manual massage and lower limb compression on symptoms of exercise-induced muscle damage in women. *Journal of Strength and Conditioning Research*. Vol. 24(11), 3157–3165

Mills, P. and Parker-Bennett, S. (2004). *Sports Massage*. Oxford: Heinemann.

Paine, T. (2007). *The Complete Guide to Sports Massage* 2nd Edition. London: A&C Black.

Monedero, J., and Donne, B. (2000). Effect of recovery interventions on lactate removal and subsequent performance. *International Journal of Sports Medicine*. Vol. 21(8): 593–597

Stasinopoulos, D., and Johnson, M.I., (2004). Cyriax Physiotherapy for tennis elbow /lateral epicondylitis. *British Journal of Sports Medicine*. Vol. 38: 675–677

Walker, B. (2007). *The Anatomy of Stretching*. Chichester: Lotus Publishing.

Ward, K. (2004). *Hands on Sports Therapy*. London: Thomson Learning.

Werner, R. (2009). *A Massage Therapist's Guide to Pathology, 4th Edition*. Philadelphia: Lippincott, Williams, and Wilkins.

Chapter

4

Advanced techniques in massage

Introduction

Once you have mastered the fundamental aspects of massage and practised your skills on a variety of athletes you can consider advanced techniques. Manual therapy techniques should be chosen and applied based on the needs of the athlete and always with their well-being as a priority.

The decision-making process should be linked directly to the techniques you will use and this needs to be fully explained to the athlete. Informed consent is a key part of providing treatment. You must consider carefully the outcomes of the techniques and how they may benefit the athlete. Supervised regular practice on a range of different athletes is needed to be successful in the module, and the revision of anatomy along with physiology and psychology should provide good underpinning knowledge.

Advanced massage techniques and their application need to be critically reasoned choices. You can support your choices by researching the recent and relevant types of evidence-based practice. Peer-reviewed journals will be a good source for this.

As with all practical skills, you should always keep up to date with the latest techniques by attending refresher courses or new programmes.

Learning outcomes

After you have read this chapter you should be able to:

- identify the reasons for applying sports massage
- discuss outcome measures
- explain soft tissue palpation
- understand the different principles of advanced massage techniques
- demonstrate different advanced massage techniques, including neuromuscular technique (NMT), muscle energy technique (MET) and soft tissue release (STR)

Starting block

Think about the therapist and the different types of massage techniques.
- What does advanced massage mean to you?
- What other knowledge would a therapist need to have before starting to apply advanced massage techniques?
- How might advanced massage techniques vary from basic massage?

Reasons for applying sports massage

Massage is a therapeutic, sensory treatment which is applied to manipulate or mobilise the soft tissues of the body. It is applied to promote the health and well-being of an athlete and to enhance performance and can be used to aid rehabilitation.

To be successful when applying advanced techniques it is important that you have a clear understanding of the musculoskeletal system, the healing process (along with knowledge relating to rehabilitation), sports injuries and sports psychology. The links to the athlete's training sessions and competition schedules, along with their current fitness levels, will all be key aspects to consider during the initial consultation.

Stop and think

Consider the different environments that you may be working in for advanced massage techniques .
- How would you prepare the different environments before an athlete arrives for treatment?
- Why might an athlete require advanced massage techniques?
- When would it be appropriate to provide advanced massage techniques?

The healing process

Before applying any massage techniques you should have a clear understanding of the healing process – this is often described as having three phases. It is important to remember that these stages often overlap and that the time limits within each one can be affected by other contributory factors.

Table 4.1: The different stages of healing

Stage of healing	
Inflammatory phase	• From approximately 0–6 days • Necessary for repair • Pain, heat, swelling, reduced range of movement (ROM) or functional activity
Proliferation phase	• Also called the regeneration phase • From approximately 3–21 days • Development of new blood vessels • Fibroblasts produce collagen fibres (type I & III) which form fibrous tissue
Remodelling phase	• Also called the maturation phase • Can take up to 1+ year • Scar tissue may develop which is less strong and less functional than original tissues

(Anderson et al. 2009)

Activity

Make a table of all the factors that you think may affect the healing process. Indicate why these would be important to consider for the athlete before applying advanced massage techniques.

Remember

When an area is injured a vascular spasm is produced which involves local vasoconstriction. This causes the blood vessels to constrict and reduces the blood flow. This can last from a few seconds up to 10 minutes. Secondly a platelet reaction occurs which provokes clotting with fibrin, this reduces the blood volume and flow to the injured area reducing blood loss at the injured site. Finally a coagulation cascade follows to aid the healing process (Anderson, 2009).

Outcome-based massage

Outcome-based massage should be a key consideration when planning treatment with the athlete. Put simply, it means you are considering what the results or outcomes of the massage will be. These 'measures' indicate a process of change from one point in time (e.g. before an intervention like massage) to another point in time (after the intervention). You must select the most appropriate outcome that supports the original aim of the treatment. For example, will the techniques be used to relieve pain, reduce scar tissue, have a restorative effect, improve range of movement (ROM) or are they going to include several outcome measures?

To achieve relevant, realistic and appropriate outcomes, it is essential that you use an 'active listening' strategy throughout the planning and treatment phases. This always starts when the subjective assessment takes place. It is about using the information provided by the athlete to give you some initial thoughts (or a hypothesis) and linking these to the objective measures. A simple step-by-step process can help you to get started:

1. Athlete presents for treatment.
2. Subjective assessment
3. Initial hypothesis
4. Objective assessment
5. Do the subjective and objective assessments support or refute your initial hypothesis?
6. Summarise and evaluate the findings with the athlete.
7. Plan and agree the advanced massage treatment or refer on if necessary.

> ### Top tip
>
> Outcome measures are usually goal and athlete focused and should be related to standards of practice. They should always be chosen to support the aim of the intervention.

Soft tissue palpation

You can improve your palpation or sensory touch skills by practising on a range of different athletes. It will help you to identify the differences between athletes and between tissues on the same athlete.

> ### Remember
>
> Always listen carefully to what the athlete tells you about any signs or symptoms they may have experienced. Remember we have two ears to listen with and one voice to speak with – use them in proportion.

These subtle differences will be sensed in a very different way by each therapist and may even change from the beginning of the treatment to the conclusion.

You should always assess the athlete **bilaterally** to avoid treating an area that may not require any intervention. Below are some basic guidelines to help you. Don't worry if some of these are not so easy to detect – practising over a period of time will develop your skills and sense of touch.

> ### Key term
>
> **Bilateral** – means on both sides of the body, e.g. left and right leg

- **Muscle tears** – Where there has been a previous grade 3 muscle tear that has since healed, the sports therapist may see or feel a noticeable dip in the normal contour of the muscle. This should be assessed by physiotherapist or doctor and imaged before massage. It may help to complete a bilateral palpation because it may be 'normal' for that individual.

- **Scar tissue** – recent scar tissue can feel firm and compact but will 'give' a little when pressure is applied. Older scar tissue can feel solid. Friction massage in the post-acute stage (when the tissue has 'plastic' properties) can help to prevent excessive scar tissue formation (Benjamin and Tappan, 2005). The friction movements break the tissue into smaller particles which can then be digested by phagocyte cells and reabsorbed into the lymphatic system. The application of any massage technique will also depend on the stage of the healing process, and with this in mind the techniques should be used to support and enhance healing.

- **Adhesions and fibrous tissue** – fibrous adhesions can affect soft tissues, especially those that are non-contractile like ligaments and tendons. These adhesions can sometimes feel gritty and can sometimes 'flick' when they are palpated, especially in a transverse direction. The application of transverse frictions separates these adhesions and, although painful, can be an effective method of managing scar tissue.

- **Fatty nodules** – these may have a corrugated feel to them when palpated. However, if the athlete has any undiagnosed lumps or swellings (especially those that have recently appeared without a reason) advise them to go to their GP.

- **Oedema** – this is an accumulation of fluid in the soft tissue which moves when palpated. When excess fluid is present the skin becomes tighter and less mobile. It may be painful when pressure is applied as the sensory nerves have increased pressure from the swelling.

- **Tension** – these can feel like small peas or pebbles under the skin. In the first instance they may be quite painful. As the area is massaged, and different pressure techniques are used, there may be a noticeable improvement for the athlete.

Activity

Practise palpation techniques on each other to locate muscles, ligaments and tendons. Identify if there are differences bilaterally and on different partners.

The principles of advanced massage techniques

Advanced massage techniques often involve the use of your arms as well as the hands and specific digits (fingers and thumbs). A reasoned choice and the safe application of these techniques, along with controlled depth and pressure, are very important.

- The thumbs – these can be used with a downward pressure, and can be angled or applied at 90°. One thumb can be used as a tool and the other to apply force and reinforce the thumb.

- The fingertips – the pads of the fingers or one digit can be used as a specific tool, or to apply force and reinforce the fingers. Ideal for smaller areas or those with little underlying adipose tissue

- The knuckles – one hand can produce a rolling movement over larger muscle groups, applied also in a sliding technique. Sometimes this is called a 'cam and spindle' technique.

- The elbow – very careful controlled pressure is needed when using the elbow as this has poor sensory feedback. The elbow can be used on larger muscle groups especially where the use of the thumb is not sufficient. The pressure from the elbow should not be used over bony areas.

- Ulnar border – this utilises the forearm and in particular the ulnar aspect which provides a wider surface area and so is ideal for large and long muscle groups.

Contraindications to advanced massage techniques include:

- acute soft tissue inflammation
- melanoma
- open wounds
- tumours
- fractures and subluxation
- cancer
- myositis ossificans
- diabetes
- thrombosis
- haemophilia
- skin diseases
- rheumatoid arthritis (Mills and Parker Bennett, 2004).

Stop and think

How can you check before applying any advanced massage techniques that there are no contraindications to treatment?

Case study

Stuart is 30 years old and plays rugby every Saturday for a local team. He visits the clinic because he sustained a muscular injury to his right anterior thigh from a collision with another player 8 days ago. He complains that when he tries to stretch the leg he has restricted movement.

Questions

1. Describe which stage of healing Stuart may present with for the thigh injury.

2. What subjective information would you need to ask Stuart?

3. Explain how the injury may feel on palpation.

4. What are the contraindications you should check for before proceeding with any treatment?

5. Establish and write down an initial hypothesis.

Neuromuscular techniques (NMT)

These are manual therapy techniques designed to influence or correct neuromuscular dysfunction. They work by the application of either a mechanical or reflex stimuli to have an influence over the neurological control of the musculoskeletal system. These techniques work by inhibiting (blocking) the neural or nerve messages from the muscles to the central nervous system (CNS) (Benjamin and Tappan, 2005; Davies, 2004).

The aims of NMT are to:

- relax muscles
- reduce tension
- relieve pain and release endorphins
- stimulate peripheral nerves.

The area to be treated should be warmed appropriately and the athlete placed in a comfortable position (and one that permits you to easily access the area to be treated). The techniques can be applied with pads of fingers, thumbs or elbow but you should always be aware of the depth that these techniques are applied with.

- Slowly palpate the area to locate the trauma or tender spot within the muscle tissue.
- Then apply gradual pressure using the pads of the fingers, thumbs or the elbow for 60–90 seconds. You should aim for deep but tolerable pressure on the specific area.

- Liaise with the athlete and advise them that the pressure may be painful at first but then should gradually subside.

- If the pain does not fade, then palpate and revisit the site up to three times, applying pressure for no more than 90 seconds.

- Keep talking to the athlete throughout the technique. Remember to ask if any pain or discomfort is fading.

Remember

If the pain does not fade during NMT, cross-fibre frictions may be applied to the area to try to loosen or free any adhesions in the tissue.

NMT can be used on a variety of conditions, including the following.

- Postural imbalance – where there is a clear identification of muscular imbalance through poor posture. This can be established during the subjective and objective assessment.

- Hypertonic muscles – these may result from a 'guarding action' over a longer period of time.

- Ischaemic effects of compression – the pressures applied have a temporary effect of reducing the blood supply to the area. Once this pressure is lifted, the blood flow is replenished, quickly removing any build-up of waste products like lactic acid.

- Musculoskeletal injury – these techniques can be used to help recovery from an injury and also to assist in the prevention of injury.

- Tender/trigger points – a trigger point is a localised spot of tenderness usually located within a tight band of muscle.

- Adhesions – any that are present within the tissues may become looser and this can improve range of movement (ROM).

The benefits of NMT include:

- restoration of musculoskeletal balance
- reduction of hypertonic muscle
- reduction of ischemia
- removal of tender/trigger points
- restoration of flexibility
- improved ROM/improved posture
- increased nutrition to muscles (Benjamin and Tappan, 2005; Davies, 2004).

Trigger points

A trigger point is a hyper-irritable neuromuscular point that is painful when compressed. It is associated with dysfunctional reflex circuits, i.e. an area that becomes so irritated that the body misinterprets the signal causing the person to feel as if the pain is coming from somewhere else. Very often an area will refer pain to a predicable spot and these are shown on trigger point charts (Niel-Asher, 2005). But each person is different and athletes will often have unique referral patterns (Archer, 2007; Davies, 2004).

These unique referral patterns can be caused by a facilitated pathway (Davies, 2004). This means a long-standing area of inflammation sends and receives nerve signals from that area; in addition any new injuries will refer pain to the old injury. Trigger point treatment can thus help to reduce facilitated pathways, returning the nerve pathways to a more normal function (Davies, 2004).

Trigger points are accumulations of waste products around a nerve receptor. They can feel like nodules or taut bands of fibres. They may form in muscles which have become overused or injured, or after surgery. They can present as a sharp pain, dull ache,

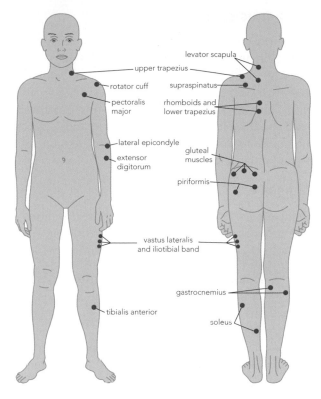

Figure 4.1: Common trigger point sites

tingling, pins and needles and hot or cold spots. Symptoms can include nausea, earache, equilibrium disturbance or blurred vision.

Deactivating trigger points

When applying pressure with the thumb on a trigger point the referral pain diminishes and the tight point of the muscle (under the therapist's thumb) softens and relaxes.

To diffuse a trigger point, static compression (pressure) is applied for 10 seconds in a pumping action while the client breathes deeply. This action 'flushes' the toxins and releases endorphins.

Ischaemic compressions

Ischaemic compressions are used in trigger point work. The aim is to deliberately increase the blockage of blood to an area so that, upon release, there will be a sudden increase in blood flow to the area. This promotes the removal of waste products such as carbon dioxide and lactic acid and supplies the necessary oxygen to help promote the recovery of the tissues (Davies, 2004).

Technique

The tissues must be warmed prior to the technique. This can be either with massage or alternative methods of pre-warming the skin and muscles.

A relaxed muscle is stretched to the point of discomfort. Initially a thumb (or strong finger) is pressed directly onto the trigger point to create a tolerably painful (7 to 8 on a client pain scale of 10), sustained pressure. As the discomfort starts to ease off, pressure is gradually increased (the other thumb or finger can reinforce and support your first thumb/ finger). This can continue for up to 1 minute. Following the treatment it is recommended to gently stretch the area to help the muscle readjust to its full length. Ice/coolant treatment can then be applied.

The first treatment should last for 1 or 2 minutes only, followed by a day of rest for the treated part. Treatment can be resumed on alternate days until the pain abates and full ROM is achieved (usually 3–10 sessions).

Remember

The visual analogue scale (VAS) is a scale from 0 to 10; with 0 being pain free and 10 being the most painful. When completing the consultation, and during the treatment, you may want to ask the athlete what level the pain is on a VAS scale, and mark this on the record card.

Frictions

Frictions are very deep penetrative and specialised techniques and are frequently used in advanced sports massage techniques when trauma has been located in muscles, tendons or ligaments. They are often used to initiate inflammation of an area in order to remodel the tissues and reduce the effects of a build-up of scar tissue.

Key term

Frictions – small concentrated movements that can be applied in a circular or transverse motion, often used to help reduce scar tissue formation

Circular frictions are performed using pads of fingers and thumbs with a small circular motion. Cross-fibre frictions (or transverse frictions) are applied transversally across the muscle fibres. The frictions should gradually increase in depth and focus wholly on the specific area to be treated.

Frictions applied correctly will allow deep penetration of the area being worked on and should produce a stretch–release effect on the tissues.

The area to be treated should be palpated and the tissue that requires friction applications specifically located by the therapist. These techniques may be painful so it is important to warn the athlete and encourage them to focus on deep breathing techniques to relieve any pain.

Technique

- Warm the tissues prior to the frictions and place the area to be treated in full stretch.
- Spread the fingers of the hand, not applying the frictions around the area of trauma.
- Locate the trauma between the index and middle fingers, or the thumb and index finger, and use them as a guider to work within the area of treatment.
- Slowly apply the frictions transversally, at a right angle to the muscle fibres being worked on. Use the pad of the thumb or finger, or the pad of the index finger with the middle finger on top for reinforcement. The latter allows a deeper pressure to be applied.
- Apply the friction using a back and forth movement. Because of the deep pressure being applied, contact with the trauma should be timed to approximately 1–3 minutes, with a total of 10 minutes per session.
- Always massage and passively stretch the area after treatment.

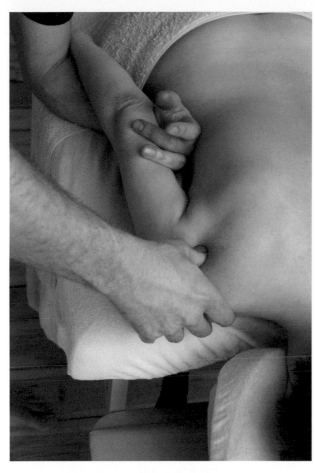

Figure 4.2: Transverse frictions technique

Soft tissue release (STR)

Soft tissue release includes a variety of techniques that, as the name suggests, 'release' soft and connective tissue such as fascia, muscles, ligaments and tendons. It is a more specific application that helps to improve the healing of certain tissues such as ligaments by separating and realigning adhesions and ultimately increasing ROM or helping to maintain stability (Sanderson, 2000). The STR techniques focus on the specific stretching and releasing of adhesions within the tissues themselves by stretching them from points located within the

adhesion. It is not just about stretching the whole length of tissues like muscles, but rather pinpointing bands of tightness and attempting to release them. Sometimes these release techniques may be very small and specific, unlike general stretching techniques.

Methods of application

Your fingers, thumbs, hands and arms can be used as effective tools in securing a **lock** on the adhesion. How they are applied will depend on the size and depth required to establish a firm and effective lock.

Key term

Lock – a lock is the firm pressure applied to an area of soft tissue to stop or limit movement

You need to have a clear understanding of the musculoskeletal system prior to treatment and in particular detailed knowledge of the fibre directions of the muscles and other soft tissues. The aim of the treatment is to apply a lock at either the distal or proximal aspect of the adherence while stretching the tissues to reduce any adherences. This lock can be achieved on small areas by using your fingers or thumbs and in larger areas with the heel of the hand or the point of the elbow.

Where there is a band of tightness, once the technique has been applied for the first time, the lock can then be reapplied by applying a new lock above the previous one. This can be repeated until the whole band of tightness has been treated. Of course, if there is just a small specific area then this can be treated on its own.

When working on the superficial fascia the lock can be applied with the pressure at an angle. However, when working on the deeper tissues, ideally the lock should be at right angles to the fibre direction of the tissues. It is important to maintain an even and consistent pressure during the lock even if you can feel the underlying tissues flickering or jumping. This will help to prevent tissue damage and bruising.

Benefits of STR

- Physical, physiological and neurological effects
- Psychological benefits which may lead to improved performance
- Decrease pain or discomfort to sensitive and hypertonic areas
- Increased local circulation
- Improvement of joint mobility
- Improvement overall soft tissue function (Sanderson, 2000).

Remember

Passive movements are performed by the therapist and not the athlete. Active movements are when the athlete moves independently of the therapist.

Types of STR

- **Passive STR** – a lock is applied and then the limb or body part is moved passively by the therapist. This method provides a good 'release' and can be very relaxing for the athlete. This passive technique usually precedes other STR techniques.

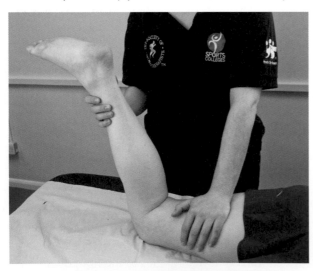

Figure 4.3: Passive STR to the hamstrings

- **Active STR** – this is a more powerful technique and should follow passive STR. Some athletes prefer this method as it allows them to control the release. This is important to bear in mind when an area is painful. Active STR involves the therapist applying the lock while the athlete attempts to stretch by moving the joint that the muscles cross. It is beneficial to the athlete if these movements replicate functional activities. For example, racquet players would benefit from movements that incorporate adduction along with protraction when releasing the pectoralis major. Thus it is important to consider the position that the athlete is placed in before you start the technique and to provide clear instructions to the athlete during the procedure.

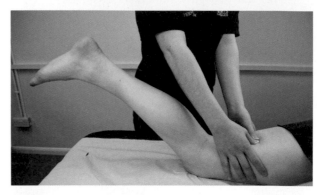

Figure 4.4: Active STR to the hamstrings

- **Resisted STR** – the principle of this technique is based upon reciprocal inhibition. For example, the hamstrings are trying to stretch and in doing so there is an isometric contraction in the quadriceps. This in turn produces an enhanced relaxation in the hamstrings. The athlete tries to produce a stretch, but the therapist provides a resistance to prevent this.

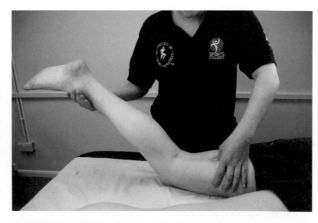

Figure 4.5: Resisted STR to the hamstrings

- **Weight bearing STR** – as its name suggests, the athlete is weight bearing during this procedure. It is an effective method of restoring full function because of the tension in the muscles and the degree of eccentric controlled contraction (Sanderson, 2000). Usually this technique should be the last stage in any treatment programme.

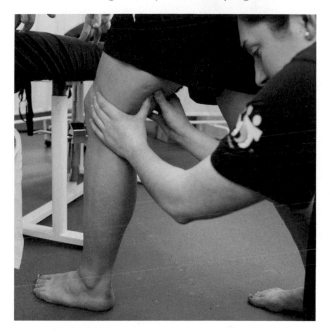

Figure 4.6: Weight bearing STR to the hamstrings

 Remember

It is good practice to explain the STR technique to the athlete, and then ask them to complete the movement before a lock is applied. You can then be sure you have explained and seen the movements before treatment.

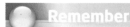 **Activity**

Practise positioning a partner and adjusting the plinth so that you could apply a variety of STR techniques for the lower leg, quadriceps, hamstrings, gluteals, upper back, upper arm and wrist.

Muscle energy techniques (MET)

Muscle energy techniques combine isometric contractions (active stretching) and passive static stretching as a means of eliciting a neurological release plus a lengthening of the soft tissue (Ward,

2004; Mills and Parker-Bennett, 2004). They can be used to mobilise restricted joints and relax hypertonic muscles while restoring muscle strength and musculoskeletal balance. These techniques can be used during the rehabilitation of injuries to help restore muscle tone and improve muscle strength and also on chronic conditions. They have several advantages, including the following.

- They can save time over deep massage.
- They often produce good results and the athlete has an active role in the procedure.
- Results are visible and easy to feel.
- They require minimal effort by the athlete to achieve results.
- Results may be clearly measured by muscle length improvement.

The disadvantages of METs include the following:

- They can be time-consuming for the therapist when working with larger teams.
- They require an extensive knowledge of muscles, origins, insertions and actions.
- They are dependent on accurate positioning of the athlete and the muscle to be effective.
- The athlete may not be able to focus and contract the target muscles.

There are two main types of METs.

1. Post isometric relaxation (PIR)

This technique works on the principle that a contracted muscle may be stretched further immediately after contraction. This is thought to be due to an inhibitory effect on the target muscle caused by the tension placed on the **Golgi tendon organ** during contraction (Ward, 2004). The contraction also creates active stretching of connective tissues. The combination of deep breaths by the athlete and mental relaxation can lead to a greater stretch.

 Key term

Golgi tendon organs – located in the tendons that attach muscle to bone. The Golgi tendon organ provides information about muscle tension which is the semi-contracted state of a muscle over an extended period

2. Reciprocal inhibition (RI)

This technique works on the principle of reciprocal inhibition. This is where an agonist muscle (prime mover) is contracted against the antagonist muscle and is inhibited to facilitate normal movement patterns. This is followed by a relaxatory period and then followed by a stretch where the muscle is stretched further.

- Passively move the joint so that the muscle is taken to the position of first resistance.
- Stabilise in this position and hold for 15–20 seconds.
- Instruct the athlete to contract target agonist muscle gently and gradually against equal resistance using about 20–30 per cent effort for about 8–10 seconds.
- Instruct the athlete to slowly relax the muscle, while inhaling deeply.
- Then ask the athlete to exhale, and while this is occurring passively move the joint beyond the new barrier, i.e. stretching the tissues.
- Stabilise this position and hold for 15–20 seconds.
- Repeat the contraction phase and the procedure again for up to as many as three or four complete cycles.

Case study

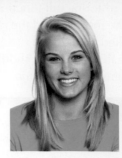

You are a self-employed therapist with a treatment room at a nearby leisure centre. Every Tuesday and Thursday you hold a 'drop in' clinic for the centre users. Amelia comes to see you. She is 18 years old and plays netball for her local team. She trains every Tuesday and Thursday evening and competes every Sunday morning. Amelia is a full-time student who works at the local supermarket every Wednesday evening and all day Saturday. She presents with a taut band of tissue in her lower left calf and also complains of aching in her right shoulder. She explains that her shoulder has become progressively worse since she started pre-season training.

On examination you note that there are active and latent trigger points on the upper back and on her lower leg.

1. Explain how you would establish that there are trigger points in the areas described.
2. Describe the treatment that you may apply, including details of the timing and frequency.
3. State how you could prepare and liaise with Amelia for treatment.
4. Identify the techniques you would use for this athlete.
5. Indicate any aftercare that you would ask Amelia to follow after treatment.

Check your understanding

1. What are the three stages of healing?
2. Why is it important that the therapist has a good understanding of these stages?
3. What are the contraindications to advanced massage techniques?
4. What is a vascular spasm?
5. State three outcome measures for advanced massage techniques.
6. Why is it important to warm tissues before applying advanced massage techniques?
7. What is an active trigger point?
8. What are the benefits of ischaemic compressions?
9. What does passive STR involve?
10. State the two types of METs .

To obtain answers to these questions visit the companion website at www.pearsonfe.co.uk/foundationsinsport

Useful resources

To obtain a secure link to the websites below, see the Websites section on page ii or visit the companion website at www.pearsonfe.co.uk/foundationsinsport.

British Journal of Sports Medicine

SportEx Health

Om Cyriax orthopaedic medicine

Sports Massage Association

Further reading

Anderson, M.K., Parr, G.P. and Hall, S.J. (2009). *Foundations of Athletic Training* 4th Edition. Philadelphia: Lippincott Williams & Wilkins.

Archer, P. (2007). *Therapeutic Massage in Athletics*. Philadelphia: Lippincott, Williams & Wilkins.

Benjamin, P.J. and Tappan, F.M. (2005). *Tappan's Handbook of Healing Massage Techniques*. New Jersey: Pearson.

Benjamin, P.J. and Lamp, S.P. (1996). *Understanding Sports Massage*. Champaign: Human Kinetics.

Clay, J.H. (2008). *Basic Clinical Massage Therapy*. 2nd Edition. Philadelphia: Lippincott, Williams & Wilkins.

Davies, C. (2004). *The Trigger Point Therapy Workbook*. Oakland: Davies & Davies.

Jarmey, C. (2003). *The Concise Book of Muscles*. Chichester: Lotus.

Mills, P. and Parker-Bennett, S. (2004). *Sports Massage*. Oxford: Heinemann.

Sanderson, M. (2000). *Soft Tissue Release*. Chichester; Corpus.

Niel-Asher, S. (2004) *The Concise Book of Trigger Points*. Chichester: Lotus.

Ward, K. (2004) *Hands On Sports Therapy*. London: Thomson Learning.

Ylinen, J. (2008). *Stretching Therapy*. London: Elsevier.

Chapter 5

Sports rehabilitation

Introduction

Rehabilitation is an ongoing process that should start from the moment of injury and continue until the athlete has returned to full participation within their sport at their original competitive level. It should be thoroughly planned and organised, allowing progression of the athlete while providing clear short- and long-term goals. Rehabilitation is about returning to full functional fitness in the safest and shortest possible time. The athlete's well-being should be the focus of the programme, and a partnership formed between the athlete and the therapist, and members of the multi disciplinary team (MDT).

Learning outcomes

After you have read this chapter you should be able to:

- understand the different stages of rehabilitation
- explain the progression of rehabilitation exercises
- discuss the factors that can affect rehabilitation
- identify a range of treatment strategies commonly used in rehabilitation.

Phases of rehabilitation

The phases of rehabilitation are linked to the healing process. There are other factors that can contribute to how the rehabilitation process progresses. You should be aware of the following for each athlete.

- The nature and mechanism of the injury.
- The structures affected as a result of the injury, e.g. hard or soft tissue (or both?).
- Other structures that may be indirectly affected as a result of injury, e.g. opposite leg or arm. Is there any evidence of compensatory mechanisms?
- The sport or activity that the athlete participates in.
- The training or exercise regimes of that individual along with the current fitness levels.
- How the athlete is managing their injury at home. Are there any social factors that need to be considered?

Rehabilitation usually takes place once the inflammation of an injured site has begun to reduce and is an ongoing process that is not always clearly bound by specific time limits.

The different types of exercise and the related muscle work used will depend on the injury, the stage of healing and short- and long-term goals.

Table 5.1 Outline aims for rehabilitation

Phase	Aims
Acute phase 0–72 hours	Control bleeding Reduce swelling Relieve pain Relieve muscle spasm Protect from further injury
Sub-acute phase 72 hrs–1 week	Disperse products of injury Promote healing Protect from further injury Restore joint mobility Restore muscle strength Maintain fitness levels Specific rehabilitation exercises Home exercise programme Gait – walking aids
Early phase 1 week plus	Regain mobility Re-develop muscle strength, endurance, extensibility Develop extensibility scar tissue Maintain fitness levels Home exercise programme – progression **Proprioception** exercises Gait – walking aids
Intermediate phase	Re-mobilise the joint Re-strengthen muscles Increase endurance, extensibility, power Increase proprioception exercises Balance and co-ordination exercises Gait – walking aids
Late phase	Re-mobilise the joint (multi joint) Re-develop muscle strength, endurance, extensibility (multi muscle) Increase endurance, extensibility, power Increase proprioception, balance, co-ordination Improve gait
Functional phase	Early functional activities (straight lines) Adjusting stride, length and pace Move to intermediate functional activities (rotating, shearing, compressing) Move to late functional activities, jumping, landing, hopping

Key term

Proprioception – the body's awareness of its position in relation to other areas of the body and whether there is movement with required effort

Acute phase

This is usually an inflammatory stage and it may be appropriate to follow the basic RICE principle when treating soft-tissue injuries:

- Rest
- Ice (if appropriate)
- Compression
- Elevation.

Before administering any first aid treatment to an athlete you must have completed an HSE-approved first aid at work qualification. The Health and Safety Executive publishes a list of approved first aid training organisations.

Remember

You must only work safely and within your scope of practice. See *Chapter 12: Ethics and safety* for more information regarding your scope of practice.

Sub-acute phase

As part of the sub-acute phase you should consider the gait cycle or walking pattern of the athlete. Some athletes may need help in readjusting their walking, running or activity styles after an injury and throughout the rehabilitation process. Gait is a sequence of co-ordinated movements that involves both single and double leg contact with a surface. The capacity to move freely or weight bear on an injured lower limb will vary. However, there are some common terms that are referred to by therapists.

- Non-weight bearing (NWB) – in both the acute and sub-acute phase the athlete may have been given axilla or elbow crutches and taught how to ambulate using them appropriately. This involves the safe use of any type of crutches from sitting to standing, standing to sitting as well as walking up and down stairs. There are different types of gait walking patterns which can be used with crutches and it will depend on the weight bearing capacity of each individual.
- Partial weight bearing (PWB) – the athlete may be using elbow crutches or a walking stick which are utilised to support the injured limb

and closely follow the pattern of normal gait, particularly when using a walking stick. As the name suggests, the athlete may be able to place some controlled weight through the limb.

- Full weight bearing (FWB) – observe the athlete walking, jogging or running and functional sporting activity. When relevant, the athlete should be able to apply their full body weight evenly during these activities. You must observe and record walking gait and stride length, and how the lower limb moves or adjusts during activity.

Remember

The athlete with a minor injury should never rely on walking aids unless advised to do so by a medical expert. Osborne and Rizzo (2003) indicate that stressing some minor ankle injuries actually helps to speed up the healing process however a comprehensive review of current evidence based literature can help the therapist's understanding (Zoch et al., 2003).

Early stages

Exercises may focus on the gentle mobilisation of the injured tissues, especially if they cross a joint or several joints. This should help to reduce pain, improve circulation and is important in maintaining range of movement (ROM) (Hengeveld and Banks, 2005). Progression can then be towards passive assisted mobilisation where the athlete may use another part of their body to help with the movement or the therapist can passively assist.

You may wish to incorporate **open kinetic chain** exercises that focus on working single muscles and single joints while remembering that keeping the rest of the body exercised is important. Fitness levels can be lost quickly during recovery, especially to uninjured tissue or the cardiovascular system, and so other forms of exercise should be considered.

Gravitational resistance can be used throughout the rehabilitation programme to progress the exercises. This can be simply achieved by changing the starting position and adjusting the length of the levers. The progressive strengthening at this stage should usually focus initially on isometric muscle work working towards isotonic exercises.

Intermediate and late stages

There should be a clear progression for the athlete, building on the previous stages. Muscle work may become more focused and the programme may now move towards developing movements that involve multiple joints and their multiple movements, with a focus on specific muscle work. Resistance work may start, particularly if it is designed to rehabilitate the specific muscles or muscle groups. The aims are to increase controlled muscular endurance, extensibility and power. Proprioception activities should be developed with the inclusion of balance and co-ordination skills.

During each stage of the programme you should introduce a variety of exercises so that the athlete is motivated. Repetitive or unappealing exercise schedules can lead to the athlete skipping key activities, possibly delaying their recovery. Exercises that incorporate the equipment that the athlete may use (such as a ball, racquet or club) can be a useful motivator. The recovering athlete may be able to undertake limited activities with the remainder of the team, especially in gym-based activities. The later stages of rehabilitation exercises should start to include simple **closed kinetic chain** movements linked to the development of strengthening muscles. Include isotonic and particularly eccentric activities while aiming to return to functional daily activities and eventually sport.

 Key terms

Open kinetic chain – a movement in which one end of the chain is open, e.g. seated knee extension

Closed kinetic chain – a movement chain in which the end of the chain is closed, i.e. in contact with the ground. Movement of one joint will produce movement of the other joints in the chain

By this stage the athlete could be fully weight bearing and initially the movements may include activities based on a linear pattern, such as walking or jogging on the spot or running at different speeds in straight lines only. When appropriate, turning activities can then be introduced and you may wish to use cones, balls and hoops to mark the exercise boundaries. As the athlete progresses, the activities may include:

- jogging in circles (from a larger to a smaller circle)
- jogging in figures of eight – reducing the size will increase the rotation forces
- side stepping
- shadowing activities with another athlete
- simple drills that incorporate rotating, shearing or compressing activities.

You should note when it is appropriate to progress the rehabilitation programme. The late functional activities should incorporate relevant activities relating to the sport which may include movements such as throwing, catching, jumping, landing, hopping and bounding. The introduction of further exercise accessories such as crash mats, benches, exercise balls and mini hurdles may add a different challenge.

Functional stage

At this stage it is necessary to introduce the patterns of movement that the athlete will undertake as part of their sporting activities. This will involve movements that work across the body rather than in a linear pattern. You should observe the active range of movements, the muscular control, the speed and agility of the response. This can be a challenging time for the athlete and they may wish to return to full competitive activities too quickly. However, programmes should progress to training with the other members of the team, or general training sessions, because at this point the athlete may be 'fit to train' but not 'fit to compete'.

Throughout rehabilitation programmes you should note that there is no single procedure that is suitable for everyone. For some athletes the rehabilitation schedule will progress in a straightforward manner and they may return to their chosen sport relatively quickly. For others this may not be the case, and you should closely monitor and record why progression is not being achieved and indicate how the programme has been amended. It may be that you have to refer the athlete to another healthcare professional who has more knowledge or experience in a specialised area, and you must refer on when necessary.

Activity

Write down the general patterns of body movement for the following activities. You should try to practise each one if it is safe to do so.

1. Backhand shot in tennis
2. Kicking a penalty in football
3. Scoring a basket in basketball

Rehabilitation programmes

You need to prepare and plan rehabilitation programmes carefully. Programmes should be based on subjective and objective assessment findings and examination and observation. Consider the **pathophysiology** of any tissues, particularly those that have been injured. In addition, all rehabilitation programmes must include progressive stages that are safe, appropriate, enjoyable and motivating for the athlete to complete.

You need knowledge of the sport that the athlete is involved in so you can establish the ultimate functional requirements of the athlete's sporting activity. This should provide clear pointers to establish the goals to work towards. For example, the functional sporting requirements of a marathon runner will be very different from those of a goalkeeper in football.

Establish with the athlete what *they* consider to be the main problem and try to address this when planning the rehabilitation programme. Ask questions to establish if there are any specific movements or activities that are causing difficulties. There should be clear communication and understanding between both parties as this helps to establish and agree goals while setting out the priorities of the treatments and programme. Close liaison with the athlete in this planning stage should lead to the development of short- and long-term goals.

Key term

Pathophysiology – the study of the changes of normal mechanical, physical, and bio-chemical functions

Short-term goals (STGs)

These should be *realistic, measurable and observable*. They may include very simple techniques that the athlete can work towards and may even be achieved in one session with the therapist. They should be followed by a clearly planned and explained homecare schedule for the athlete to undertake between sessions.

Short-term goals (STGs) are established to help plan treatments, very often to meet some previously established outcome measure and as steps towards meeting the long-term goals. For the therapist they can help to prioritise treatment and establish the effectiveness of the planned programme.

In some cases it may be that the therapist links these STGs to communicate therapy goals with other members of the multi disciplinary team or even to refer the athlete on to other health care professionals.

Long-term goals (LTGs)

These are the goals that may take several sessions or even weeks and months for the athlete to achieve. Ideally, one constant long-term goal (LTG) may be for the athlete to return to full functional fitness and competition. LTGs should link directly with the STGs and be listed in an order of priority. They may include the re-setting of both types of goals during the rehabilitation programme when targets may or may not be achieved.

Remember

The short- and long-term goals should be reviewed each time the athlete visits the therapist. Ongoing evaluation is essential as rehabilitation programmes may need to be amended to meet the needs of the athlete and their recovery.

Activity

Give some examples of short- and long-term goals during the early stage of rehabilitation in a netball player who is recovering from a grade 2 sprained ankle.

Grading muscle strength

There are different methods of assessing and grading muscle strength (Clarkson, 2000). The Medical Research Council or Oxford grading system is one measure of muscle strength you can use to help determine and record a client's muscle strength. It is linked to each athlete's age, fitness level, and any previous injury to an area. You must have a good knowledge of the musculoskeletal structures in order to identify the muscle groups and specific muscles. (See *Chapter 1: Functional anatomy* for more detail on the musculoskeletal system.) A fully fit athlete may be expected to score 5/5.

1. Flicker of movement
2. Through full range but not against gravity
3. Through full range against gravity
4. Through full range with some resistance
5. Through range with full resistance

Activity

In pairs, identify how the Oxford scale might vary for the following:

- 2 days after a first degree muscle strain to the quadriceps
- 21 days after a cast is removed for a fractured wrist
- 14 days after a grade II ankle sprain.

Repetition maximum (RM)

This is a method of measuring the strength and endurance of a muscle or group of muscles, usually to test isotonic muscle strength (Fleck and Kraemer, 2004). A therapist may refer to a 1RM – this is the *maximum* amount that an individual can either push or lift in one movement; this is not an ideal measure for the untrained or rehabilitating athlete. Instead a suitable alternative may be a 5 or 10RM and should focus on the athlete completing the movement in a controlled and pain free way. However, it should be challenging and demanding enough to permit progression, ideally working towards the point of minimal discomfort for the athlete. *Chapter 7: Training and conditioning* covers muscle work and range of movement in more detail.

Progression

Treatment and exercise progression should be based on the healing of tissues and linked to the pathophysiology of the injury. Progression should be based around different programmes of current evidence-based treatments and exercises which support the whole process of rehabilitation. Progression will not depend on one factor alone, and the therapist needs to observe and liaise closely with the athlete throughout the programme. When deciding if it is relevant to progress the exercises, the following questions need to be considered before progression continues.

- The quality of movements – are they performed in a slow and controlled manner?
- Is the athlete free from pain?
- Can the movements be repeated?
- Are the movements consistent and smooth?
- What is the feedback from the athlete?

Controlling movements

You can draw on very simple techniques to progress exercises and improve mobility and strength. These can be used as indicators to see if it is relevant to move on to the next stage of rehabilitation. The *speed* and *control* of the movements during specific exercises gives some indication of how the athlete is responding to the agreed goals. The same exercise can be progressed by adjusting or adding the following.

1. Slowing the movement to establish the control of the activity.
2. Adding a series of 'stops', 'holds' and 'starts' at different points within the range of movement.
3. Using different starting positions – half lying, sitting, standing.
4. Utilising different grasps – under grasp, over grasp, pushing off.

The size of the base

The base is the area that is in contact with a surface. This could be the floor, a chair, a stool or even a plinth. Generally the wider the base or the more contact the body has with a base the more stable the athlete will be. If the athlete has a support surface, if the therapist lowers this support surface, it can make exercises progressive and challenging.

The height of the base

An athlete who sits on a chair with both feet placed on the ground will move from sitting to standing more easily (requiring less effort and muscular control) than a client moving from sitting on a lower stool to standing. The hardest of all will be moving from a low bench to standing. Therefore, simply by altering the height of the support surface, a progression can be achieved.

> ### Activity
>
> Stand up and put both your feet very close together. Then sit on a chair and compare the areas that are in contact with a surface. Which one is most stable?
>
> Devise a series of starting positions, one for the shoulder and one for the knee, that include the different types of starting positions that a therapist could use when planning exercises for different stages of rehabilitation.

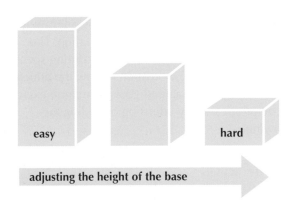

adjusting the height of the base

Figure 5.1: Progressions from sitting to standing

The effects of gravity and progression of exercise

Gravity and its role in rehabilitation exercise is a useful tool that the therapist and the athlete can use to their advantage. When this is linked to the starting position of the exercises, or even treatment, gravity has a very important role to play (Houghlam, 2005).

Exercises are easiest to complete when the centre of gravity is lowest; this is usually a lying position

either on the floor or on a plinth. In this position there is a *horizontal* transference of weight and the athlete can use this in order to move limbs or other parts of the body while they are fully supported.

To progress exercises the therapist may decide to use a diagonal transference of weight *across* gravity, for example by placing the injured area in a position of 45° to the floor. This could be achieved simply by altering the starting position from supine lying to side lying.

The next stage is to work *against* gravity. This usually means working the injured limb at 90°, where there is a vertical transference of weight. This can be achieved in a sitting or standing position and will depend on the injured aspect of the body.

> ### Activity
>
> 1. Devise two exercises for the following areas: shoulder, wrist, abdomen, gluteals, thigh and ankle.
> 2. Indicate the easiest starting position for each exercise where there are minimal effects of gravity.
> 3. Explain how each exercise can be progressed from the initial starting position of gravity eliminated to working across gravity and finally to against gravity.
>
> Think carefully about the starting position and any resources or equipment required for you to complete this activity.

Assistance

Exercises can also be progressed by removing any assistance (e.g. the therapist no longer performs passive movements on the athlete) and moving on to passive, active assisted movements, and then finally on to active resisted movements.

During rehabilitation, other forms of assistance may be employed, e.g. the therapist may recommend the use of wall bars to assist in supporting movements, crutches may assist with gait, or even the athlete's own body (e.g. their arms or legs) may be used initially to help with a movement. When starting balance training, the athlete may use their arms or legs to help maintain balance. A client sitting on a Swiss ball for the first time may need to use their feet and arms to stabilise their position; a client who is recovering from an ankle injury may use their arms or wall bars to maintain their balance if standing on their injured ankle. Simple progressions when safe to do so may be made by asking the athlete to perform a movement without the use of these supports.

Adding resistance

Resistance can be provided in different ways during the progression of exercises. Gravity, as already discussed, can be used extensively. This, along with specific movements and physical accessories, can add interest and challenges to the athlete's programme. Accessories can include dumbbells, beanbags, hoops, sticks, thera-bands or even something related to the athlete's sport, possibly a racquet, golf club, football or a hockey stick.

Remember
Progression can sometimes be achieved be adjusting by the length of the lever.

When *not* to progress exercise

You must know when *not* to progress treatment and exercise, and to recognise when the athlete is not progressing in the rehabilitation programme. This may be resolved by simple adjustments of the goals that accurately reflect the athlete's needs but it may be that the programme needs to be thoroughly revised and amended.

Lack of progression may be due to other factors such as:

- disruption to the healing process
- unclear communication between the therapist and the athlete
- athletes not following homecare routines and guidance accurately
- overambitious planning of STGs
- incorrect selection of treatment and exercises
- changes in the athlete's exercise or training patterns
- plateauing of the recovery process
- other illness or injury.

Factors that can affect rehabilitation

Poor rehabilitation can cause a series of problems for all types of athlete. You must be aware of the factors that can adversely affect progression and return to full functional activities. Functional activities are not those movements related just to sport, but include movements that your client may undertake as part of normal daily living. This can involve what seems like simple activities such as climbing stairs, sitting down, or even getting dressed. When an athlete is recovering from injury, these activities can be challenging and consider them as a key part of the rehabilitation programme.

Activity
With a partner, compile a table of functional activities linked to a sport of your choice. Think of activities:
- that a client might undertake during a normal competition match or game from arriving at the club to after a match
- that a client might undertake when at home.

Poorly planned and organised rehabilitation can lead to the following problems.

- **Longer healing time** – if an athlete tries to undertake too much too soon, then the healing process may be disrupted and could lead to more scar tissue formation. This has subsequent problems on range of movement and activity. This can cause longer term problems for the athlete and may lead to chronic conditions which are more difficult to address and may cause them considerable discomfort.
- **Prone to re-injury** – an athlete who does not adequately recover from injury and progress through the appropriate activities in the stages of recovery may find that the same injury recurs.
- **Longer to return to active sport** – most athletes will want to return to sporting activity as quickly as possible. However, the process of recovery from injury linked to the rehabilitation process should be carefully controlled and monitored. Very often your client will reach the stage where they are 'fit to train' but not 'fit to compete'.

- **Psychological effects** – these can be key factors in the recovery process and should be considered carefully as part of the rehabilitation programme. For some athletes in team sports, or those who have severe or chronic injuries that are recovering over a period of months, the rehabilitation process can seem a negative process. Some athletes miss the camaraderie and involvement of frequent training schedules and competition. You may want to set treatment or exercise schedules for when the team are together.

- **Social effects** – athletes who have family commitments may not be able to take part in normal family or social activities because of their rehabilitation programme. For athletes who live alone this can be an isolating time and sometimes simple day-to-day activities like writing or getting dressed can become a major difficulty.

- **Weight changes** – those who are confined to limited activity may gain weight due to lack of exercise and movement, or experience general lethargy. Consider how general fitness may be maintained during the whole of the recovery process.

- **Financial worries** – these are often a reason why athletes want to return to training and competition too soon, especially if their sport rewards them financially for their skills and participation.

The 'population' of your athletes?

As a therapist, you will work with different athletes and with different *populations*. You must think about how to manage the different athletes' rehabilitation programmes and establish how maintenance of the fitness levels will be addressed. Some specialist populations may include:

- mature or elderly athletes
- disability athletes
- children or youths (See *Chapter 12: Ethics and safety* page 163 for more information about working with young people and children.)
- pregnant athletes.

Stop and think

Are there any other factors that may affect the rehabilitation process? Think about both team and individual sports.

Treatment strategies commonly used in rehabilitation

Any treatments that are applied to promote healing and enhance recovery must be based on current evidence and you should always justify your choices and decisions and agree these with your client.

Usually thermal therapy will work in a continuum from coolant through to heat, and this will be linked directly to the stage of injury and recovery. Ideally, in the acute stage, the tissues may need to be cooled, but as the injury starts to repair the emphasis can move towards heat therapy (Anderson et al., 2009).

Thermal therapy

Thermal therapy includes heat and coolant treatment, which can be applied during the rehabilitation process. You need to understand the physiological effects of both heat and coolant treatments, the different methods of application and how to use these safely and appropriately. When using different forms of thermal therapy consider:

- the area to be treated – remember that fat (adipose tissue) insulates against heat/cold; skin will respond to thermal treatment in approximately 6–8 minutes, muscles may take much longer (Palmer and Knight, 1992)
- the intensity of the application – some thermal treatments will generate a cooling or heating effect very quickly while others may be slower
- the timing or duration of the treatment – for some coolant treatments the optimum overall application time may be no longer than 20 minutes.

Cryotherapy (cooling)

The principle of cryotherapy is to reduce blood flow by constricting the blood vessels. Coolant therapy works not by causing the area to become cold, but by drawing heat away from the injured tissues, which ultimately has a cooling effect (Merrick et al., 2003). Cooling is beneficial and often used in the early stages of injury because it:

- reduces swelling
- has an **analgesic** effect
- reduces capillary blood flow therefore there is less swelling
- causes local vasoconstriction, which slows down the blood flow to the area
- controls oedema
- reduces muscle spasm
- reduces metabolism in the tissues and so lessens the risk of extending tissue damage because of lack of oxygen.

Key term

Analgesic – a method of providing pain relief

Some coolant treatments are inexpensive and can be used at the pitch side in a first aid capacity. Other treatments may be used more appropriately in a clinical based situation. Remember that each method has its own advantages and disadvantages and the selection of any treatment should always be based on the needs and the best interests of the athlete. All treatments should be explained and agreed with your client prior to application.

Remember

The Lewis Hunting Reaction occurs when a coolant such as an ice pack is applied to the skin. The blood vessels in that area vasoconstrict (narrow) and then after a short period of time (about 10–12 minutes) they vasodilate (widen). This protects tissues from prolonged cooling and prevents hypoxia – a lack of oxygen to the area.

Remember

Minimising bleeding to the injured area may help to speed up the healing process of soft tissue.

Different types of coolant include the following.

- **Simple ice pack** – ideally this should be crushed ice placed in a thick plastic bag that is secured so that when the ice melts the water does not flood the treatment area. This can then be wrapped in a damp cloth and applied to the area to be treated. Alternatively, an ice bag can be used; these can be partially filled with crushed ice and cold water so that the bag 'conforms' and fit snugly around the treatment area.

- **Gel pack** – these are placed in the freezer for at least 24 hours to cool and then wrapped in a damp cloth before being applied to the skin. Sometimes these gel packs do not easily conform to the area being treated. Some gel packs are designed to be multi-use and can be heated to use as a warming treatment.

- **Coolant bandage** – this involves the application of a specially purchased bandage and an accelerator. The bandage is applied in the normal way and can be left in place for up to 2 hours. After use the bandages can be cleaned and re-impregnated with a chemical coolant accelerator for future use.

- **Coolant sprays** – these can be used on localised areas and can produce a very quick cooling effect. There is a danger that the spray, if not directed carefully, can enter the eyes or other tissues and it should never be applied to or sprayed near broken skin.

- **Disposable ice pack** – as its name suggests, this is a single-use item, activated by twisting the ice pack. This initiates a chemical reaction within the sealed pack that immediately produces a cooling effect. A barrier should always be applied to the skin before application as these packs can cool the tissues very quickly.

- **Ice block** – cold water can be placed either in a styrofoam cup or a specially purchased plastic container and placed in the freezer. This can then be used to apply localised cooling to most areas of the body. When using this method a barrier of oil is usually placed on the skin first to prevent ice burns.

- **Cryocuff** – this treatment simultaneously combines the coolant therapy with compression. The container is filled with iced water and attached to a cuff. There is normally a selection of different cuffs which are designed to contour and fit different areas of the body like the knee, ankle, shoulder or elbow. Once applied to the area the cuff inflates rapidly to produce the desired effect. This can be a quick and effective method of treatment, especially in a clinical situation. There are also alternative branded products such as Game Ready which combines intermittent compression along with ongoing circumferential cold therapy.

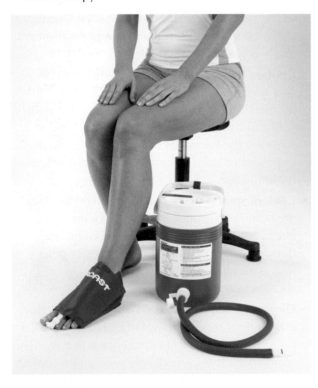

Figure 5.2: A cryocuff – what do you think are the advantages and disadvantages of using this method of treatment?

Thermal therapy in the sub-acute phase

After the acute phase the treatment may then move on to a combination of heat and coolant therapy. At this point the tissues may still have some swelling but there should be no inflammatory heat being produced from the area and bleeding should already have been controlled. The physiological effects of the sub-acute phase include

Top tip

Ice baths work on a different principle where the athlete submerges their body (usually up to the waist) in a bath of iced water. The benefits are thought to be achieved by the general reduction of metabolism after a strenuous event followed by vasodilation and the removal of waste products to promote recovery once blood flow is increased. However, some research indicates that this may not always be the case (Howatson et al., 2009; Crowe et al., 2007). McAuley (2001) and Bleakley et al., (2004) suggest that further research is needed to establish an evidence base on the use of ice baths when used in sport. The sports therapist needs to read the current evidence-based research regarding cryotherapy and think about how this may affect their practice.

Remember

Never apply a cooling medium such as an ice pack directly on the skin – always have a barrier such as a damp cloth between the skin and coolant.

the absorption of swelling and removal of any debris (Anderson et al., 2009). There will also be the growth of new blood vessels along with the development of fibrous repair tissue. The emphasis of treatment changes in this phase and the key aims of treatment are now to:

- disperse the products of inflammation
- promote the healing process
- protect the part from undue stress
- begin early mobilisation of the joint
- begin early tone work for muscles.

Contrast bathing

The ice treatment used in the acute phase is now replaced with contrast bathing, where the injured limb is subjected to alternating periods of hot and cold. This causes an opening and closing of the blood vessels, which aids the re-absorption of the swelling and promotes healing. Although contrast bathing refers to the submersion of tissues in water, sometimes the location of a recovering injury will not permit this, e.g. thigh, shoulder, and so you may have to use coolant packs and warmed gel packs, to provide the alternating cooling and heating effects.

When preparing for this treatment the temperatures should ideally be:

- cold water or application approx 10°C to 18°C (50°–65°F)
- warm water or application approx 38°C ° to 44°C (100°–111°F).
- in sub-acute conditions one method is to base the treatment on a variable time frame which alternates in the first cycle between 75 per cent in cold water immersion and 25 per cent in warm water immersion.

It is important that during the treatment an *active range* of movements is continued while the injured part is immersed.

Table 5.2: Contrast bathing

Modality cold/hot	Cycle 1	Cycle 2	Cycle 3
Cold	3 or 4 mins	2 mins	1 min
Hot	1 min	2 mins	4 mins
Cold	3 or 4 mins	2 mins	1 min
Hot	1 min	2 mins	4 mins
Cold	3 or 4 mins Finish on COLD	2 mins Finish on COLD	1 min
Hot			4 mins Finish on HOT

(Anderson et al. ,2009)

Heat therapy

When there is clear evidence that the tissues are positively responding to treatment, you may want to include the use of heat therapy (Anderson et al. 2009). The physiological effect of superficial heating produces a localised rise in skin temperature, but remember that underlying deeper tissues are warmed to a lesser extent because of the insulating effects of subcutaneous fat. Superficially there will be local vasodilation of the skin's blood vessels which will help to remove waste products from the area, removing any oedematous swelling by the increased blood flow as well as having a sedative effect on the sensory nerve endings.

Heat therapy will have a pain relieving effect and can help to decrease any muscle spasm or 'guarding' that may have occurred as a result of the injury and lack of mobility during the earlier phases and treatments. The warming of the tissues can therefore also help to increase the range of movement (ROM) at the joints in combination with the improved extensibility of warmed muscular tissue (Anderson et al., 2009). Different types of heat modalities include the following.

- **Gel pack** – some of these packs can be heated by immersing in warm water and gently heating through before application. Others can be heated in a microwave. It is essential to read the manufacturer's instructions on each pack as they vary in how they may be safely heated.
- **Paraffin wax bath** – the use of paraffin wax baths in gently heating tissues can be a useful modality in the clinical setting. They are ideal for warming the hands and feet although the wax can be applied to joints by 'layering' the wax during application. Once applied, the treatment area is usually wrapped in plastic and then covered with towels in order to maintain the gentle heating effect. The wax can remain on the treatment area for up to 20 minutes.

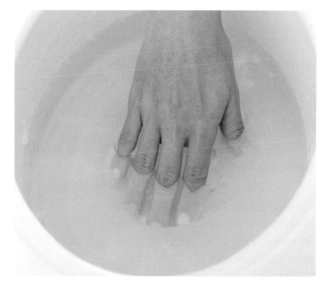

Figure 5.3: A paraffin wax bath. What contraindications might you need to consider when using a wax bath?

- **Hydrocollator heater and packs** – this method of heating is achieved by moist or wet heat, with specialised pads immersed in boiling water when placed in a heater. On application the pads must be wrapped in plastic and towels to allow diffuse heat and to prevent scalding the athlete.

- **Radiant heat lamps** – these are small portable lamps that can be placed on a table or moveable stand. Take care that the portable lamp is placed on a safe base, and that the lamp is positioned at the correct distance from the area to be treated (usually no nearer than 18 inches) with the heat directed at the treatment area at an angle of 90° for maximum absorption of the heating effects. Lamps should never be placed directly over an athlete.

- **Heat gels/sprays/creams** – these are superficial warming products that are not generally used by therapists in sports settings, although some athletes use them to warm tissues or as a temporary method of pain relief. They can be purchased as non-prescription items at chemists.

Remember

Heat therapy can be applied by using very simple measures like an insulated hot water bottle, a warm bath or even a warm hydrotherapy pool.

Thermal therapy safety precautions

- Always complete a skin sensitivity test using small test tubes, one with warm water another with cold, and test the area to be treated.
- Never apply a cooling or heating medium directly to the skin.
- Explain to the athlete that they need to tell you if the skin is feeling too cold or hot.
- Never leave on for more than 15 minutes in any one hour.
- Check the tissues throughout the treatment.
- Never apply for longer than is necessary – this can cause more damage to tissues.
- Always check the circulation during treatment (fingers and toes).
- Always ask the athlete how the area feels regularly throughout the thermal treatment.

Dangers of thermal therapy

- Super cooling the skin
- Skin burns both by heat and coolant
- Fainting
- Fat necrosis (death of tissue)
- Severely reduced circulation
- Increased bleeding to an area

Remember

The athlete should never lie with any body weight on a coolant or heat modality. This can cause permanent tissue damage.

Contraindications

Before applying any treatment check for any contraindications to the treatment. Good practice indicates that before each treatment you should re-establish with the athlete that there have been no changes in their health since their previous session.

Table 5.3: Contraindications to thermal therapy (× = contraindicated, N/A = not applicable)

Contraindications	Cryotherapy	Heat therapy
Skin infections	×	×
Varicose veins	×	×
Haemorrhage	×	×
Broken skin – cuts or abrasions	×	×
Impaired circulation	×	×
Lack of thermal sensitivity	×	×
Cardiac patients	×	×
High or low blood pressure	×	×
Recent deep vein thrombosis	×	×
Diabetes	×	×
Allergy to wax	N/A	×
Open wounds	×	×
Raynaud's disease	×	×
Nerve palsy	×	×
Lupus	×	×
Acute inflammation	N/A	×
Advanced arthritis	N/A	×

Hydrotherapy

The benefits of rehabilitating and exercising in water are well documented. Hydrotherapy can provide support to the injured athlete while helping to maintain mobility, improve strength and cardiovascular fitness. The depth of the water can add greater demands to an activity while reducing weight bearing stresses on joints. Bouyancy aids such as floats, flippers or paddles can be used within a rehabilitation programme to support or add resistance (Marra et al., 2001; Belza et al., 2000; Spitzer-Gibson and Hoeger, 2003). Now consider the following points.

- What are the benefits of **hydrotherapy exercises** in sports rehabilitation?
- What are the beneficial effects of exercising in the pool?
- Give examples of hydrotherapy exercises that could be introduced to the different stages of a rehabilitation programme.

Resources

The resources that are available will vary from one therapist and sports club to another. It may be that there is only a small rehabilitation area available with limited space and equipment; other therapists may have access to a fully equipped gym and a wide range of resources. The adaptable therapist will learn to work with their knowledge in a variety of settings and where possible establish links to share or hire resources that may help in the planning of rehabilitation and delivery of programmes. Equipment may include thera-bands, trampettes, balance pads, crutches or heat packs. For some clubs the access to larger resources like gyms with fixed weights, fitness testing equipment or hydrotherapy pools may be very limited or at amateur level may rely on the player using their own personal gym membership. In these cases the therapist may have to provide specific advice for the athlete to access such resources in their own time in order to follow a programme.

Key term

Hydrotherapy exercises – these are completed in water or a pool. They can be used in all the stages of injury and can add variety to the recovery programme

Activity

Compile a list of the different types of equipment and resources that a freelance therapist could use as the basis of a 'rehabilitation resource toolkit'.

Case study

A professional football player has suffered a ruptured Achilles tendon while playing. The team's doctor has arranged for him to have surgery and has indicated that recovery could take five to eight months, with the fear that his football career could be finished.

1. At the time of the injury, describe which structures may have been injured and how this affects the functional ability of the player.
2. Outline the short- and long-term goals of a treatment plan in the sub-acute stage of injury.
3. Explain which treatments you could apply in the early stages of injury and how they will support the rehabilitation process.
4. What factors will you need to consider when deciding if progression of the rehabilitation programme is appropriate?
5. Devise an exercise plan for the functional stage of rehabilitation for this injury.

Check your understanding

1. What are the key aims of rehabilitation programmes?
2. State four reasons why a client may not progress in their rehabilitation programme.
3. Name three coolant treatments and state one advantage of each.
4. Explain when heat treatments would be beneficial in a rehabilitation programme.
5. List five contraindications to thermal therapy.
6. What are the specialist populations that a therapist may work with?

7. Which ways can the therapist use gravity in exercises?
8. Why are short- and long-term goals important in rehabilitation?
9. List six different types of equipment the therapist could use in an exercise programme.
10. Name three examples of functional sporting activities.

To obtain answers to these questions visit the companion website at www.pearsonfe.co.uk/foundationsinsport

Useful resources

To obtain a secure link to the websites below, see the Websites section on page ii or visit the companion website at www.pearsonfe.co.uk/foundationsinsport.

British Journal of Sports Medicine

Virtual Sports Injury Clinic

SportEx Medicine

Further reading

Anderson, M.K., Parr, G.P. and Hall, S.J. (2009). *Foundations of Athletic Training* 4th Edition. Philadelphia: Lippincott, Williams & Wilkins.

Belza, B., Topolski, T., Kinne, S., and Patrick D. (2000). Adherence to Aquatic Exercise Programs: Results from a Randomised Clinical Trial. *The Gerontologist*. Vol. 56(9), 1–22

Bleakley, C., McDonough, S., Mc Auley, D. (2004). The Use of Ice in the Treatment of Acute Soft-Tissue Injury; A Systematic Review of Randomized Controlled Trials. *The American Journal of Sports Medicine*. Vol. 32(1), 251–261

Clarkson, H.M (2000) *Musculoskeletal Assessment; Joint Range of Motion and Manual Muscle Strength 2nd Edition*. Philadelphia, Lippincott, Williams & Wilkins

Comfort, P. and Abrahamson, E. (2010). *Sports Rehabilitation and Injury Prevention*. Chichester: Wiley Blackwell.

Crowe, M.J., O'Connor, D. and Rudd, D. (2007). Cold Water Recovery Reduces Anaerobic Performance. *International Journal of Sports Medicine*. Vol. 28(12), 994–8.

Fleck, S. and Kraemer, W. (2004) *Designing Resistance Training Programmes*. Champaign: Human Kinetics

Gormley, J. and Hussey, J. (2005). *Exercise Therapy Prevention and Treatment of Disease*. Oxford: Blackwell.

Gotlin, R.S. (2008). *Sports Injuries Guidebook*. Champaign: Human Kinetics.

Hengeveld, E., Banks, K., (2005) *Maitland's Peripheral Manipulation*. London: Elsevier Butterworth Heinemann.

Higgins, R., Brukner, P. and English, B. (2006). *Sports Medicine*. Oxford: Blackwell.

Houghlam, P.A. (2005) *Therapeutic Exercises for Musculoskeletal Injuries* 2nd Edition. Champaign: Human Kinetics.

Howatson, G., Goodall S., Van Someren, K. A. (2009) The Influence of Cold Water Immersions on Adaptation Following a Single Bout of Damaging Exercise. *European Journal of Applied Physiology*. Vol. 105, 615–621.

Marra, D.J., Boda, W., Gale, J.B., McHugh, E., Burch, D. (2001). Effects of Vertical Water Exercise on Selected Muscle Strength Measures Among women Age 24–55 years. *Research Quarterly for Exercise and Sport*. Vol. 72(1), A–22.

Merrick, M.A., Jutte, L.S. and Smith, M.E. (2003). Cold Modalities With Different Thermodynamic Properties Produce Different Surface and Intramuscular Temperatures. *Journal of Athletic Training*. Vol. 38(1), 28–33.

McAuley, D. (2001). Do Textbooks Agree on Their Advice on Ice? *Clinical Journal of Sport Medicine*. Vol. 11(2), 67–72.

Osborne, M. D. and Rizzo, T.D. Jr. (2003). Prevention and Treatment of Ankle Sprain in Athletes. *Sports Medicine*. Vol. 33(15), 1145-1150.

Palmer, J.C., Knight K.L. (1992). Ankle and Thigh Skin Surface Temperature changes with Repeated Ice Pack Application. *Journal of Athletic Training*. Vol. 27, 138.

Shultz, S.J., Houghlam, P.A. and Perrin, D.H. (2005). *Examination of Musculoskeletal Injuries*. Champaign: Human Kinetics.

Spitzer-Gibson, T.A., Hoeger, W.K. (2003) *Water Aerobics for Fitness and Wellness* 3rd Edition California: Thomson Wadsworth.

Thygerson, A.L. (2008). *Injury Prevention* 3rd Edition. Sudbury: Jones & Bartlett.

Zoch, C., Fialka-Moser, V., Quittan, M. (2003). Rehabilitation of Ligamentous Ankle Injuries: A Review of Recent Studies. *British Journal of Sports Medicine*. Vol. 37, 291–295.

Chapter 6

Fitness testing for sports therapy

Introduction

Fitness testing is commonly undertaken in the professional practice of sports therapists. Whether you are doing basic field-based testing, or more complex testing in a laboratory environment, you need to be familiar with the purpose, process and methods of interpreting each of the tests that you will do. The work of a sports therapist in fitness testing is multifaceted. You will need to be able to measure the fitness levels of the most unconditioned of individuals, as well as being able to measure the match fitness of a higher level athlete prior to a return to competition. You may even need to take elite athletes through functional specific tests to help monitor performance. In any of these scenarios, you must treat each client with the same professionalism and cater for their individual needs. In the later stages of functional rehabilitation and return to competition, fitness testing is as important as your physical assessment skills in the early stages of injury.

Throughout this chapter you will learn about the different fitness tests that are commonly used in sports therapy and how to conduct them.

Learning outcomes

After you have read this chapter you should be able to:

- know the rationale for fitness testing within sports therapy
- know the process of fitness testing a client
- know a range of fitness tests that are commonly used within sports therapy
- be able to conduct the different fitness tests that are commonly used within sports therapy
- be able to interpret the results of different fitness tests that are commonly used within sports therapy.

Starting block

Think about the following clients: a 70-year-old retired IT worker, an 18-year-old female football player and a 30-year-old male volleyball player with a history of knee injuries. What would you need to take into consideration about each of these clients before deciding which fitness tests they should do?

The rationale for fitness testing within sports therapy

Fitness tests are used in sports therapy for different reasons including:

- providing motivation for clients when they see improvement in fitness levels during later stages of rehabilitation or post-rehabilitation
- designing fitness training programmes
- providing baseline fitness levels from which you can monitor improvement
- monitoring progress and adapting fitness training programmes
- checking the functional ability of clients post-rehabilitation and pre-match
- as part of a team selection process
- to make players aware of their responsibility to other team members.

The process of fitness testing a client

Although all fitness tests are different there is a general process that you can follow. This process allows the client to gain confidence in you and the process that you are going to follow. The process is as follows.

To be completed prior to the testing session

1. Address health and safety issues within the testing environment (including calibrating and testing any equipment).

2. Prepare a results recording sheet.

To be completed on first meeting the client at the testing session

3. Introduce yourself and reassure the client about the process they are about to go through – this is particularly important if it is a client who has been passed on to you and this is your first meeting.

4. Complete a pre-test medical questionnaire. This is essential to identify any relevant or important health issues that could be possible contraindications to testing.

5. Complete informed consent with the client. This provides the permission from the client to conduct the fitness testing. You should not do any fitness testing without the client's consent and you should make it clear to the client that they can stop the testing at any point. Allow the client the opportunity to ask any questions.

Top tip

When preparing to test your client, prepare the environment so that it causes minimal embarrassment, for example check that there is an appropriate amount of privacy in the testing setting. This is particularly important when conducting girth measurements and skinfold measurements.

To be completed at the testing session for each fitness test

6. Reassure the client about the individual test.

7. Explain what you are testing and why.

8. Explain the method of testing.

9. Explain the equipment.

10. Allow the client the opportunity to ask any questions.

11. Carry out the test.

12. Collect the results.

13. Interpret results.

14. Give feedback (verbal).

15. Ask the client if they have any questions.

16. Give feedback (written), providing recommendations for maintenance or improvement (as appropriate for the client).

When fitness testing clients, it is important to make sure that you select normative data that is specific to your client group. Using generic norm data with specific groups (e.g. gender, age and high level athletes) can lead to invalid conclusions regarding the fitness status of the client. For examples of normative data, see Heyward (2010); Heyward and Wagner (2004) and Hoffman (2006) (see Further reading page 92 for more information).

Top tip

When providing recommendations to maintain or improve fitness test results, always give specific recommendations that are geared towards the needs of the client rather than providing general statements.

Health- and skill-related fitness tests commonly used within sports therapy

Fitness means different things to different people. The term fitness can be defined as the ability of an individual to meet the demands of their environment and can be separated into health-related components of fitness and skill- or sport-related components of fitness. Health-related components of fitness are those that, if improved, would have overall benefits for health (but can also influence sport performance in athletes) whereas

skill or sport-related components of fitness are those that, if improved, will have overall benefits for sports performance. With the nature of skill- or sport-related components of fitness, they are largely specific to the sport you participate in. For example, a 100 m sprinter needs to have more of a **mesomorph** body composition (health-related component of fitness) and high levels of speed, power and a fast reaction time (skill-related components of fitness) to be a successful sprinter, but the components of fitness required to be a successful alpine skier would be very different. Table 6.1 defines the different components of fitness and identifies their associated fitness tests.

Key term

Mesomorph – a body type that is characterised by heavy, toned muscle content. The shoulders are broad, the thorax is large, the waist is quite slender and the abdominal muscles are defined

Table 6.1: Components of fitness and their associated tests

Component of fitness	Definition	Associated fitness tests
Agility	The ability to move and change direction quickly while maintaining control of the movement	Illinois agility run
Body composition	The ratio of fat mass to lean tissue in the body	Skinfold testing Bioelectrical impedance Body mass index Girth measurements Waist to hip ratio Height and weight charts
Cardiorespiratory endurance	The ability to provide and sustain energy aerobically	Resting heart rate Blood pressure Lung function testing Multi-stage fitness test Yo–Yo endurance test 1 mile walk test Astrand–Rhyming test Ventilatory breakpoint test Cooper 12 minute run 1.5 mile run test Laboratory-based maximal oxygen uptake testing
Flexibility	The range of movement at a joint	Sit and reach test Goniometry
Muscular endurance	The ability of a muscle or muscle group to sustain repeated contractions over an extended period of time	1 minute press-up test 30 second sit-up test
Power	The ability to generate and use a large amount of force in a short space of time	Vertical jump Standing broad jump Wingate test
Speed	The maximum rate at which a person can move over a given distance	Sprint tests
Strength	The amount of force that can be produced by a muscle or muscle group during a maximal contraction	Hand grip dynamometer 1 repetition maximum (1RM) Isokinetic dynamometer (measures strength and power)

Top tip

As well as the different fitness tests above, you should always consider using postural assessments at the start of your fitness testing session if it is a new client. This is because postural deviations may be a consideration of (or contraindication to) some of the different fitness tests that you decide to use.

Conducting fitness tests

Throughout this section, you will be introduced to the different protocols for the different fitness tests. When familiar with the testing protocols, try to conduct the tests with a friend or colleague who can act as your client. While you are still learning the practical skills try to conduct the tests in the presence of an appropriate professional (such as a sports therapist or lecturer).

Measuring resting heart rate

Resting heart rate is commonly measured using heart rate monitors or by palpating key sites. The two most common sites that are palpated are the carotid site and the radial site. The pulse rate is measured by lightly placing the tips of the second and third digits at either the carotid or radial site and then counting for a number of seconds to attain the pulse rate. The pulse rate in beats per minute is calculated by multiplying the number of beats by the required amount (e.g. if you have counted the number of beats in 10 seconds, you will have to multiply this by 6 to calculate the number of beats per minute).

Resting heart rate is best measured in the morning on waking. If this is not practical, allow your client 5 minutes rest prior to measuring their heart rate. Generally, the lower the resting heart rate (within safe limits), the less work the heart has to do to pump the same amount of blood around the body, indicating greater cardiorespiratory endurance. The average pulse rate of a 'normal' individual will fall in the range of 60–80 beats per minute. Be aware of the conditions of **bradycardia** and **tachycardia**. Bradycardia is often seen in high level endurance athletes (Hood and Northcote, 1999) whereas tachycardia can be caused by stress (Hassan et al., 2009) or poor diet or can be a sign of underlying cardiac conditions. Remember that some

medication such as beta blockers can decrease resting heart rate (Dufour Doiron, Prud'homme and Boulay, 2007).

Measuring blood pressure

- Using a mercury sphygmomanometer, blood pressure should be taken in the sitting position from the right arm. The arm should be relaxed resting on a flat surface.

Key terms

Bradycardia – a resting heart rate below 60 beats per minute

Tachycardia – a resting heart rate greater than 100 beats per minute

- Wind the arm cuff around the upper arm and place the bell of the stethoscope in the antecubital space over the brachial artery (see Figure 6.1).
- Inflate the cuff to a pressure of 200 mmHg and then adjust the valve so that the air is released gradually from the cuff.
- Listen through the stethoscope until the first sound or vibration is heard – this is the systolic blood pressure (SBP). As the cuff pressure decreases the sounds will cease – this point denotes the diastolic blood pressure (DBP). The sounds that you are listening for are known as the **Korotkoff sounds**.
- Repeat this process for the left arm and check for bilateral differences.

A tutorial on the measurement of blood pressure is available from the British Hypertension Society (refer to the *Useful resources* section on page 92).

Because blood pressure alters throughout the day, you should not classify your client as either **hypertensive** or **hypotensive** on the basis of a single measurement. Take a number of different measurements at different times to get a clearer picture. You should remember that, as a sports therapist, it is outside the limits of your practice to make a medical diagnosis. If you think that a client may have problems with their blood pressure, you should refer them to their GP.

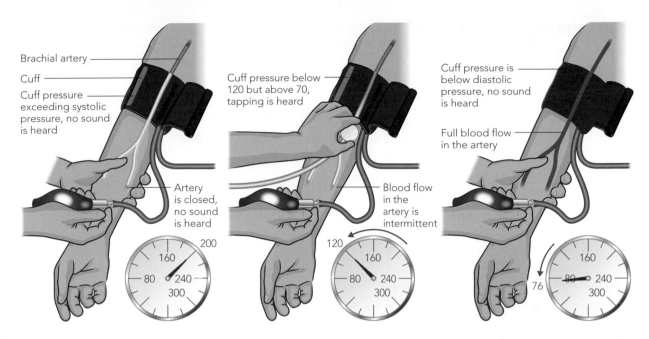

Figure 6.1: Process of blood pressure measurement

Key terms

Korotkoff sounds – the sounds that sports therapists listen for when measuring blood pressure using a mercury sphygmomanometer and stethoscope

Hypertension – high blood pressure of 140/90 mmHg or above

Hypotension – low blood pressure 90/50 mmHg or below

Measuring body mass index

Body mass index (BMI) is used to identify people who have particular body composition/health issues (e.g. overweight, obese). Unfortunately, the BMI is not the most accurate measure as it does not take into account key variables. For example, some rugby players may weigh a lot but most of their weight could consist of muscle (not fat). However, the BMI is still widely used but is best used in conjunction with other methods of body composition assessment.

BMI is calculated using the following calculation:

$$BMI = \frac{weight\ (kg)}{height\ (m)^2}$$

BMI can also be calculated using a nomogram (see Figure 6.2). Find your height and weight and using a ruler and a pencil join the two points to find your BMI.

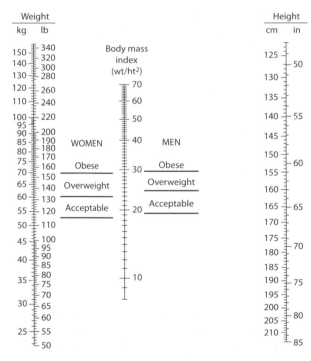

Figure 6.2: Body mass index nomogram. What is your BMI value from the nomogram?

(Reprinted by permission from Macmillan Publishers Ltd: International Journal of Obesity (Bray, G.A. (1978). Definition, measurements and classification of the syndromes of obesity. Vol. 2, 99–112), copyright (1978).)

Height and weight charts

Height and weight charts can be used to give an indication of people's body composition, but they don't give any indication of body fat and don't take into account factors such as activity levels or sports played. Therefore it is not recommended for use with elite athletes. Your rating is recorded by finding your height and weight on a chart (see Figure 6.3) and marking the point where the two values meet.

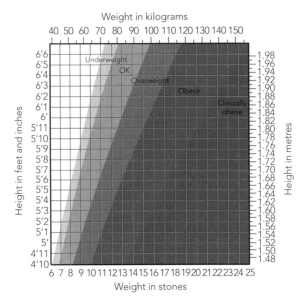

Figure 6.3: Height and weight charts. What do you think are the limitations of using these charts with athletic populations?

Waist to hip ratio

Waist to hip ratio can be used to look at the distribution of body fat in the upper and lower body. As the test looks at the amount of fat around the abdominal area, it can identify people who are at risk of conditions such as obesity, hypertension, coronary heart disease and diabetes. A high waist to hip ratio could lead to other lifestyle assessments.

Use an anthropometric tape to take measurements at the narrowest part of the waist (just above the iliac crest and across the umbilicus) and the widest part of the hip (normally the widest point just above the level of the greater tronchater). After taking your measurements, complete the following equation:

$$\frac{waist\ circumference}{hip\ circumference}$$

Be careful when taking this measurement as it is prone to invalidity and poor test/retest reliability if an inexperienced therapist is taking the measurement. There are sources of errors if standard tape measures are used rather than specific anthropometric tapes.

Girth measurements

Girth measurements assess the size of body areas and give an indication of fat distribution. The following recommendations are for clients so that they can effectively complete testing if they are:

- fully recovered from previous exercise.
- fully hydrated
- fully voided
- suitably attired:
    - males: running shorts or swimwear are ideal
    - females: running shorts and a sports top that exposes the abdomen and shoulders are ideal.

Some clients may not be comfortable with these guidelines, so a loose fitting T-shirt which can be lifted to allow access to measurement sites is acceptable. If you are working with a client of the opposite gender, have an assistant of the same gender as your client working with you. If you are working with a minor make sure a parent or other chaperone is present.

When taking girth measurements follow the steps below and use the information in Table 6.2.

- Approach the participant from the side.
- Hold the end of the anthropometric tape in your left hand and the stub of the anthropometric tape in your right hand.
- Pass the stub of the tape around the body segment and then pull to the appropriate tension.
- Make sure that the tape stays at 90° to the long axis of the segment.
- There should be no visible indentation of the skin – if this occurs then your measurement is too tight.
- For torso measurements, the measurement should be taken at the end of a normal expiration.

Table 6.2: Girth measurement sites

Girth measurement	Location	Body position
Chest	At mid-level of the sternum	Arms abducted slightly
Waist	Narrowest circumference between thorax and pelvis	Arms folded
Hip	At the level of maximum posterior protuberance of buttocks	Relaxed, feet together
Upper arm	Mid acromiale–radiale level	Arm abducted slightly, elbow extended
Forearm	Maximum	Shoulder slightly flexed, elbow extended
Mid-thigh	Mid trochanterion–tibiale level	Weight equally distributed
Calf	Maximum	Weight equally distributed

Skinfold calliper based assessment of body fat

Injured athletes can face the problem of an increase in body fat levels. In order to help them regulate this, you need to be able to take appropriate skinfold measurements. These identify the amount of subcutaneous fat.

To complete this test you need a set of skinfold callipers, such as the Harpenden skinfold callipers. You need plenty of experience to be able to take reliable measurements so follow the protocol below step by step. Inexperienced therapists struggle to correctly identify the measurement sites, are unfamiliar with the use of skinfold callipers and can struggle to correctly grasp a skinfold. All of these factors can lead to issues with inter-observer reliability (when body fat is measured by different researchers), test/retest reliability and invalidity.

It is important that you are supervised while you are learning to use the callipers to increase the accuracy of measurement. Several protocols can be used but

the one below is the Durnin and Womersley (1974) four site method used to predict a client's body fat levels.

Protocol

1. Measurements should be taken on the right hand side of the body unless there is a tattoo or skin condition that dictates otherwise.

2. Carefully identify, measure and mark the skinfold sites:

   a triceps – vertical skinfold exactly halfway between the olecranon process and acromion process. The arm should be held freely by the side of the body

   b biceps – vertical skinfold on the anterior surface of the upper arm at the midpoint between the anterior axillary fold and the antecubital fossa

   c subscapular – oblique skinfold taken 1 cm below the angle of the scapula (at approximately 45°). This should follow the natural line of the skin

   d suprailiac – taken diagonally, directly above the iliac crest.

3. Grasp the skinfold firmly and confidently between thumb and index finger.

4. Gently lift the skinfold.

5. Keep the fold elevated while you take the measurement.

6. Place the jaws of the callipers approximately 1 cm below the thumb and index finger and slowly release the pressure.

7. Make a note of the reading.

8. Open the jaws of the calliper before removing it. Close the jaws gently.

9. Take each measurement three times in sequence (TRI, BI, SS, SI x 3 in that order).

10. Work out the mean result for each of the sites. Add the four means together to get a total skinfold in mm.

11. Convert your result in mm to a body fat percentage using a skin fold conversion table. Refer to the Useful resources section on page 92 for more information.

Bioelectrical impedance

Bioelectrical impedance body fat monitors usually take the form of a small battery operated unit that has electrodes and adhesive pads that are attached to specific sites on the body, with the client lying in a supine position. Other bioelectrical impedance units include hand-held measures or measures that are similar to conventional weighing scales and can be bought from many chemists.

Bioelectrical impedance works on the premise that fat free mass conducts electricity, so the greater the conduction of the electrical signal, the greater the level of fat free mass (Heyward and Wagner, 2004). Bioelectrical impedance units can give you information about your client including fat mass, fat weight, water content, lean tissue and basal metabolic rate depending on the equipment that you are using.

Lung function testing

Lung function testing assesses the effects of conditions such as asthma and **dypsnea**.

The most popular measure of lung function is peak flow which can be measured using a simple peak flow meter (e.g. the Mini Wright peak flow meter). Other measures such as **forced expiratory** volume (FEV$_1$), **forced vital capacity** (FVC) and **forced expiratory ratio** (FER) can be measured using a microspirometer. Although sport performance is not greatly limited by peak flow, it is a good measure of health-related fitness.

Key terms

Dypsnea – difficulty in breathing or shortness of breath

Forced expiratory volume – the percentage of vital capacity that can be expired in one second

Forced vital capacity – the amount of air that can be forcibly expired following a maximal inspiration

Forced expiratory ratio – the ratio of FEV$_1$ to FVC

Protocol for measuring peak flow using a peak flow meter

1. Ensure the meter reads zero.
2. Ask the client to stand (unless disabled or carrying an injury that can prevent this).
3. Client takes a deep breath.
4. Client places the peak flow meter in their mouth and seals their lips tightly around the mouthpiece.
5. The client must breathe out as hard as they can; leaning forward towards the end to ensure

any residual volume is expelled. This will take approximately 1–2 seconds.

6. Repeat this three times.
7. Record the score and compare it to the norm data (peak flow norm data charts can be downloaded in .pdf formats for both adults and children (see Useful resources page 92 for more information)

FVC, FEV$_1$ and FER can be measured using a microspirometer in the same way as peak flow is measured using the peak flow meter. FVC normally ranges from around 4–5 litres in healthy males (although values of approximately 6 litres are not uncommon in very tall males), and around 3–4 litres in healthy females. A FER value of around 80–85 per cent is normally observed in healthy individuals, but in clients with severe asthma or emphysema, values have been known to be as low as 40 per cent (Sonne and Davis, 1982).

Cooper 12 minute run

The Cooper 12 minute run is a maximal test which estimates **VO$_2$ max** using the distance that a client can run as the estimation. Once you have recorded the distance, use the following equation to calculate the VO$_2$ max value:

$$(distance\ (m) - 504.9)\ /\ 44.73$$

The distance achieved can be compared to a table of norm data to give an overall rating for different clients to monitor progress.

Although this test can be completed on a treadmill, either use a 400 m running track or use cones to mark out a 400 m track. Completing the test in this way has reported a correlation of 0.90 between VO$_2$ max and the distance covered (Cooper, 1968).

Key term

VO$_2$ max – the maximum amount of oxygen that can be taken in and utilised by the body in one minute; while breathing at sea level. VO$_2$ max is expressed as either absolute or relative values

Protocol

1. The client must run as far as they can. Walking is allowed if they cannot run but they should be reminded that the aim of the test is to cover as much distance as possible. Keep going for

the full 12 minutes. This test is a maximal test therefore if the client does not put in the full effort, the results will be invalid and unreliable.

2. Work out VO_2 max using the equation above and compare the distance to a table of norm data to get a rating.

Multi-stage fitness test

The multi-stage fitness test (MSFT) is often used to predict VO_2 max by fitness professionals because it requires limited equipment, is easy to administer, and is suitable for the assessment of large numbers of clients.

Several studies have shown it to be a reliable measure of VO_2 max, although some have shown that the MSFT does underestimate VO_2 max levels when compared to laboratory-based treadmill measures (Cooper, Baker, Tong, Roberts and Hanford, 2005; McNaughton, Hall and Cooley, 1998). While the MSFT is capable of measuring changes in aerobic fitness levels in those who have lower levels of baseline fitness, there are some questions as to whether the MSFT is sensitive enough to assess the development of aerobic fitness in clients who are high level performers (Svensson and Drust, 2005).

Protocol

1. Client performs a short warm-up (not too vigorous as the early stages of the test will be similar to a warm-up pace).
2. Client stands on the start line and, on hearing the triple beep, runs to the other line 20 metres away. They must reach the line on or before the single beep that determines each shuttle. The client must make sure that they do not get ahead of the beep, so they should try to match their running speed to it.
3. Client continues to run each stage until volitional exhaustion. You should monitor their achievement of each stage, giving them two verbal warnings if they fail to achieve a stage. The third time that the client misses a stage, they should be withdrawn from the test.
4. On completion of the test, compare the stage they have achieved to relevant norm data to get a prediction of their VO_2 max.
5. Compare the predicted VO_2 max to relevant norm data.

1.5 mile run test

The 1.5 mile run test is used as an indicator of aerobic endurance in athletes where there is not a varying pace during the event. It is not widely used with athletes who play team sports due to its poor replication of match conditions.

It is best conducted on an indoor athletics track or on a dry outdoor athletics track. Alternatively, mark out a distance in an indoor sports hall and monitor the performance that way.

Protocol

1. Perform a warm-up and complete appropriate stretching.
2. Client runs a distance of 1.5 miles in as fast a time as possible.
3. Record the time taken to complete the test.
4. Compare the result to relevant norm data.

1 mile walk test

You will also work with clients who need to go through lower intensity tests (such as clients who have high levels of obesity). This test is best performed on a dry level surface (such as an athletics track or a sports hall).

Protocol

1. Perform a gentle warm-up before the start (including the stretching of any relevant muscles or muscle groups).
2. Client walks 1 mile in as fast a time as possible.
3. Record the time taken in minutes.
4. When the client crosses the finish line, measure the pulse rate for 15 seconds and then convert to beats per minute by multiplying the 15 second count by 4.
5. Use the formula on page 86 to predict **absolute VO_2 max** ($l.min^{-1}$).

Key terms

Absolute VO_2 max – maximal oxygen consumption expressed as $l.min^{-1}$

Relative VO_2 max – maximal oxygen consumption expressed relative to the client's body weight in kg and measured in $ml.kg.min^{-1}$

VO$_2$ max = 6.9652 + (0.0091 × wt) − (0.00257 × age) + (0.5955 × gender) − (0.2240 × t) − (0.0115 × HR)

Where:

wt = body weight in lbs

age = age in years

gender = 0 if female, 1 if male

t = time in decimal minutes

HR = heart rate (beats per minute).

1. Convert the absolute VO$_2$ max to **relative VO$_2$ max** using the following equation:

   Relative VO$_2$ max = [(absolute VO$_2$ max × 1000) ÷ weight in kg]

2. Compare the calculated VO$_2$ max to relevant norm data.

Remember

If you have a client who is unable to run, the 1 mile walking test is a more suitable test option than running-based tests.

Laboratory-based assessment of oxygen uptake

When working with professional team sports players or Olympic endurance athletes laboratory-based testing may be necessary. Oxygen uptake is measured in laboratories using specific protocols and either treadmills, cycle ergometers or rowing ergometers. You need knowledge of protocols such as the Bruce protocol, the Astrand-Rhyming test, YMCA cycle ergometer protocol and the ACSM cycle ergometer protocol. (See the *Further reading* list on page 92 and Reilly and Eston (2008a), Reilly and Eston (2008b) and Hoffman (2006) for details of these protocols.)

Stop and think

What do you think are the advantages and disadvantages of laboratory-based and field-based methods of assessing VO$_2$ max tests? Why do you think it is important for a sports therapist to have an understanding of types of testing?

Sit and reach test

The sit and reach test is the most commonly used test of lower back and hamstring flexibility. It is useful for therapists working with athletes who are prone to hamstring injuries, e.g. football players and sprinters. To complete this test, you need a sit and reach box.

Top tip

When conducting the sit and reach test, use observation techniques to try to identify any areas of tightness in the client (e.g. in the lumbar region or in the hamstrings).

Protocol

1. Client performs a gentle warm-up (including stretches of relevant muscles) prior to the test.

2. Removes shoes and sits on the floor. Client extends legs so that they are flat on the floor and the soles of the feet are in contact with the sit and reach box.

3. Places one hand on top of the other and reaches forward slowly, in one complete movement, moving the slider as far forward as they can. Advise the client not to bounce.

4. Repeat three times.

5. Record the best score and compare it to relevant norm data.

NB With this type of norm data, the toe line counts as 0. Therefore, moving 1 cm past toe line counts as +1, moving to 1 cm before the toe line counts as −1cm

Goniometry

Goniometry is a direct measurement of flexibility that can be conducted at any joint using a goniometer. This can provide precise measures of flexibility but sometimes it is difficult for an inexperienced therapist to precisely locate the joint centre so supervision while learning is recommended.

Protocol

1. Place the centre of the goniometer at the axis of rotation of the joint.

2. Line the arms of the goniometer up with the long axis of the specified bones when the limb/section is in its normal resting position.

3. Perform the desired movement.

4. Measure the range of movement using one of the arms on the goniometer. The range of movement is recorded in degrees on the angle gauge.

Once you have recorded the range of movement at a given joint, you can compare the angle to the norms for different joints that are included in *Chapter 2: Introduction to sports injury and assessment*.

Hand grip dynamometer test

The hand grip dynamometer is designed to take a direct measurement of maximal static strength that can be generated by the client. It is important to understand that, although it measures maximal static strength, the results of this test should not be used as an indicator of strength in other areas. Ensure you follow the set protocol to avoid injury.

Protocol

1. Client performs a gentle warm-up before the start (including stretching of relevant muscles and muscle groups).

2. Holds dynamometer in hand with display facing away from body.

3. Starting with dominant hand, client grips dynamometer maximally. Client must not bend arm and must stay standing up straight.

4. Repeat test three times on each hand, alternating between hands after each attempt.

5. Record the best result from dominant and non-dominant hand.

6. Compare the result to relevant norm data.

1 repetition max (1RM)

The 1RM measures the amount of weight that a muscle or muscle group can move in a single maximal contraction. This test is performed using a fixed resistance machine, but a better way is to use free weights as these do not provide any assistance and give a more accurate measurement of unassisted 1RM. If you use this type of test using free weights, ensure that there are adequately capable spotters so that you do not put your client's safety at risk. The 1RM can be adapted for use with most muscles or muscle groups.

Protocol

The protocol below is for a 1RM using a fixed resistance machine testing the quadriceps muscle group on a leg extension exercise.

1. Client performs a gentle warm-up before the start (including stretching of relevant muscles and muscle groups).

2. Sits with legs in position on leg extension with arms either crossed over chest or behind back with hands palm down on bench. Client should not hold onto bench as this can give extra leverage and can lead to invalid and/or unreliable results.

3. Make a decision at an initial load close to, but below, the client's maximum capacity.

4. Client attempts to lift, breathing out on exertion so as not to increase blood pressure too much.

5. If lift is successful, progress to next weight up (range between 1 5 kg). If lift is unsuccessful, drop to weight below (same range).

6. Always leave a rest interval of between 1 and 5 minutes before client attempts to lift heavier weight.

7. The results of the 1RM are recorded in two ways:

   a an absolute value of the weight lifted

   b relative to the mass of the client. To calculate this, you divide the 1RM result (in kg) by your client's body weight (in kg) and use relevant norm data to interpret the result.

30 second sit-up test

This tests the local muscular endurance of the abdominal muscle group. To perform this test, you need a stopwatch to time 30 seconds and a mat for your client to reduce the risk of any back injuries.

Protocol

1. Client performs a gentle warm-up before the start (including stretching of relevant muscles and muscle groups).

2. Lay the client down on the mat, with their knees flexed at right angles.

3. Place hands next to head with elbows pointing forwards.

4. Perform as many sit-ups as they can in 30 seconds.

5. Record the number of complete sit-ups in 30 seconds.

6. Compare the result to relevant norm data.

1 minute press-up test

This tests the local muscular endurance of the muscle groups in the upper arms and chest.

Protocol

1. Client performs a gentle warm-up before the start (including stretching of relevant muscles and muscle groups).

2. Client positions themselves on the mat. Hands should be shoulder width apart and back straight (the adapted position for females can be used as part of this test).

3. Place a fist on the mat under the chest of the client (positioning the fist under the forehead may be more appropriate for females but monitor the press-up technique if this version of measurement is used).

4. One press-up is classed as the client going down, their chest touching the fist of the tester and then returning to the starting position.

5. At the end of the test, compare your client's result to relevant norms.

Sprint tests

This type of test is often used in the later stages of functional rehabilitation, post rehabilitation or as part of a pre-match fitness test. The example below is the method for completing a 30 m sprint test. It can be completed using a results recording sheet and a stopwatch or specific testing equipment such as the Newtest powertimer that measures your speed using light gates and sends the data to a handheld PDA device. The latter can often be a more valid and reliable measure as human error is removed from the testing procedure.

Protocol

1. Mark out a 35 m line with markers at 0 m, 5 m and 35 m.

2. Client performs a gentle warm-up before the start (including stretching of relevant muscles and muscle groups).

3. Using a flying start (a sprint from 0–5 m to ensure that acceleration does not invalidate the results), client sprints as hard as they can from start to finish.

4. Start timing at the 5 m mark (start line) and stop timing at the 35 m mark.

5. Record the time in seconds and compare the results to relevant norm data.

Standing vertical jump

The standing vertical jump test indicates the amount of power that can be generated by an individual by looking at how far the centre of mass moves. It is often best performed using a vertical jump mat as this method measures how far the client's centre of mass moves. Alternative methods (such as using millisecond jump mats) can be susceptible to measurement error as the vertical jump height is determined by the period of time that the feet are not in contact with the floor. This means that a client who lifts their feet further from the floor (for example by bending their legs) could get a higher vertical jump score while actually having less movement of the centre of mass. This test is often used in late stages of functional rehabilitation, in post rehabilitation or as part of a pre-match fitness test.

Protocol

1. Client performs a gentle warm-up before the start (including stretching of relevant muscles and muscle groups).

2. Attach vertical jump mat around waist.

3. Wind dial until string is tight.

4. Switch jump mat on.

5. Client jumps vertically as high as they can (ask them not to jump horizontally off the mat as this will invalidate the result).

6. Perform the test three times.

7. Record your client's best result and compare the result to relevant norm data.

Standing broad jump

The standing broad jump is another indicator of power in the legs, but it is used with athletes where horizontal distance is more important than vertical distance.

Protocol

1. Client performs a gentle warm-up before the start (including stretching of relevant muscles and muscle groups).
2. Stands with feet shoulder width apart and with toes behind line.
3. Client jumps as far forward as possible.
4. Do this three times.
5. Record the client's best result and compare their score to relevant norm data.

Laboratory-based assessment of power

As with oxygen uptake, there are laboratory-based measures of power, with the most common being the Wingate test. (See the *Further reading* list on page 92 and Hoffman (2006), Maud and Foster (2006) for details of the Wingate testing protocol.)

Illinois agility run

The Illinois agility run measures speed and agility over a prescribed course. It is suitable for any sports that require the ability to move, and change direction, quickly. It is used post rehabilitation to gain a baseline measure from which the client can be monitored. Adapted versions of this test (or at least the figure of eight movements) can also be used in pre-match fitness tests.

Protocol

1. Mark out an area 10 m in length.
2. Place four flexible markers 3.3 m apart.
3. Client performs a gentle warm-up before the start (including stretching of relevant muscles and muscle groups).
4. Lies prone, head to start line, hands beside their shoulders.
5. Client runs the course as fast as they can (as shown in Figure 6.4).
6. Record the client's time and compare to relevant norm data.

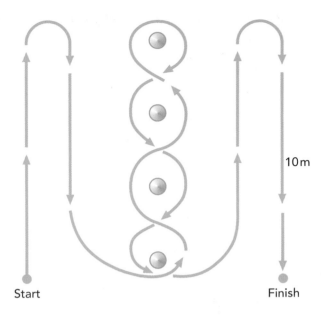

Start   10 m   Finish

Figure 6.4: Illinois agility run test. It is important for the client to familiarise themselves with the test procedure prior to this test being administered. Why do you think this is?

> **Stop and think**
>
> When selecting fitness tests, select tests that are valid, reliable and objective. When working in healthcare settings, why is it important to consider these different factors?

Special considerations when working with elite athletes

When working with elite athletes it is likely that you will be doing much more functional and sport-specific testing and will have to compare the elite athlete to their previous fitness levels or the fitness levels of others in their team or event as the standard norm data is based on general population norms rather than norms for elite athletes. Although norm data is available for a range of different tests, it is beyond the scope of this chapter to include norm data for all relevant populations. Use sport-specific texts and testing manuals for particular groups of elite athletes (e.g. Reilly and Eston, 2008a, Reilly and Eston, 2008b).

Remember

Always seek out sport-specific norm data if you are going to use norm data to assess the fitness test results of elite athletes.

Pre-match fitness testing

When a client is injured or has been through their rehabilitation programme and is returning to full fitness, they will ask 'When can I play again?' You can answer this question by using a pre-match fitness test.

It can take place at any time up to the day of an upcoming game or event so that you can accurately judge the ability of the client to participate.

Pre-match testing may involve some of the fitness test movements that are performed in different tests (such as vertical or horizontal jumps, short sprints, figure of eight runs) and will be aimed at the injury site and types of movements or skills (such as tackling or heading a football) that the client will have to perform in the upcoming game or event.

Interpret the results of fitness tests

Most commonly, fitness test results will be interpreted against norm data. However, this may not always be appropriate (if you are working with an elite athlete) so the following methods are used to interpret different fitness test results:
- comparison of current fitness levels to previous fitness levels
- comparison of immediate post rehabilitation fitness levels to pre-injury fitness levels
- comparison of results to similar athletes that are performing at similar levels (such as teammates who play in the same position in the same team).

Top tip

Comparing current fitness levels to previous fitness levels can be good for the motivation of the client as it avoids negative social comparisons and gives them a clear indication of how much better they are getting.

Case study

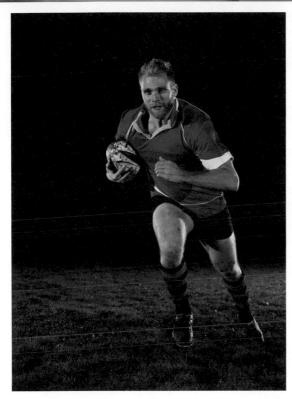

A rugby fly half was cut down by an ankle injury. At the time it was seen as potentially career threatening. His dislocated and broken right ankle required surgery and meant that he could not play rugby for 6 months. One of the biggest problems for the support staff who worked with him was to make sure that, first, he would be fit and ready to return to playing rugby without a serious risk of re-injury and second to get him back to a level of fitness that would allow him to play at pre-injury levels again.

As a sports therapist, you would need to play an active role in this rehabilitation period. The fitness testing elements that have been discussed throughout this chapter play an integral part during the later stages of functional rehabilitation or in post rehabilitation.

1. What are the special considerations when working with this type of client?

2. What fitness tests do you think would have been appropriate to assess this client and why?

3. How would it be best to interpret the different fitness test results with this client?

Check your understanding

1. Why do sports therapists use fitness testing?

2. What is the process of fitness testing a client and why is it important to follow this process?

3. What are the main fitness tests associated with sports therapy?

4. What are the validity and reliability issues commonly associated with body composition assessment?

5. Why is pre-test screening important in fitness testing?

6. Why is consent important in fitness testing?

7. How do you interpret the results of different fitness tests in sports therapy?

8. How can the results of fitness tests guide your post rehabilitation work with clients?

9. What are some of the special considerations for testing elite athletes?

10. What is the purpose of a pre-match fitness test?

To obtain answers to these questions visit the companion website at www.pearsonfe.co.uk/foundationsinsport

Useful resources

To obtain a secure link to the websites below, see the Websites section on page ii or visit the companion website at www.pearsonfe.co.uk/foundationsinsport.

Video tutorial on blood pressure measurement from Aberdeen Medical Faculty

British Hypertension Society

Harpenden Skinfold Calipers – downloadable client sheets, a skinfold calculation Excel® file and information on body composition assessment using Harpenden Skinfold Calipers

Podcasts from the National Strength and Conditioning Association on fitness testing, training and programming

Mini Wright Peak Flow Meter – information relating to the importance of peak flow and the norm data for peak flow levels in adults and children

Sports Fitness Advisor – how to design a battery of physical fitness tests

Further reading

American College of Sports Medicine (2006). *ACSM's Guidelines for Exercise Testing and Prescription* 7th Edition. Philadelphia: Lippincott, Williams & Wilkins.

Brummit, J. (2010). *Core Assessment and Training.* Champaign: Human Kinetics.

Cooper, K.H. (1968). A means of assessing maximal oxygen uptake. *Journal of the American Medical Association,* Vol. 203, 201–204.

Cooper, S-M., Baker, J.S., Tong, R.J., Roberts, E., and Hanford, M. (2005). The Repeatability and Crtierion Validity of the 20m Multi-Stage Fitness Test as a Predictor of Maximal Oxygen uptake in Active Young Men. *British Journal of Sports Medicine,* Vol. 39, 216–222.

Dufour Doiron, M., Prud'homme, D., and Boulay, P. (2007). Time of Day Variation in Cardiovascular Response to Maximal Exercise Testing in Coronary Heart Disease Patients Taking a Beta-Blocker. *Applied Physiology, Nutrition and Metabolism,* Vol. 32, 664–669.

Durnin, JVGA, Womersley, J. (1974). Body fat assessed from total body density and its estimation from skinfold thickness: measurements on 481 men and women aged from 16 to 72 years. *British Journal of Nutrition.* Vol. 32, 77–97.

Hassan, M., Mela, A., Qin Lin, M.S., Brumback, B., Fillingim, R.B., Conti, J.B., and Sheps, D.S. (2009). The Effect of Acute Psychological Stress on QT Dispersion in Patients with Coronary Artery Disease. *Pacing and Clinical Electrophysiology,* Vol. 32, 1178–1183.

Heyward, V.H. (2010). *Advanced Fitness Assessment and Exercise Prescription* 5th Edition. Champaign: Human Kinetics.

Heyward, V.H. and Wagner, D.R. (2004). *Applied Body Composition Assessment.* Champaign: Human Kinetics.

Hoffman, J. (2006). *Norms for Fitness Performance and Health.* Champaign: Human Kinetics.

Hood, S., and Northcote, R.J. (1999). Cardiac assessment of veteran endurance athletes: a 12 year follow up study. *British Journal of Sports Medicine,* Vol. 33, 239–243.

Maud, P.J. and Foster, C. (eds.) (2006). *Physiological Assessment of Human Fitness* 2nd Edition. Champaign: Human Kinetics.

McNaughton, L., Hall, P., and Cooley, D. (1998). Validation of Several Methods of Estimating Maximal Oxygen Uptake in Young Men. *Perceptual and Motor Skills,* Vol. 87, 575–584.

Reilly, T. and Eston, R. (eds.) (2008a). *Kinanthropometry and Exercise Physiology Manual: Tests, Procedures and Data. Volume One: Anthropometry* 3rd Edition. London: Routledge.

Reilly, T. and Eston, R. (eds.) (2008b). *Kinanthropometry and Exercise Physiology Manual: Tests, Procedures and Data. Volume Two: Physiology* 3rd Edition. London: Routledge.

Sonne, L.J., and Davis, J.A. (1982). Increased exercise performance in patients with severe COPD following inspiratory resistive training. *Chest.* Vol. 81, 436–439.

Svensson, M., and Drust, B. (2005). Testing Soccer Players. *Journal of Sports Sciences,* Vol. 23, 601–618.

Ward, K (2004). *Hands on Sports Therapy.* London: Thomson Learning.

Winter, E.M., Jones, A.M., Davison, R.R.C., Bromley, P.D. and Mercer, T.H. (eds.) (2006a). *The British Association of Sport and Exercise Sciences Sport and Exercise Physiology Testing Guidelines Volume 1: Sport Testing.* London: Routledge.

Winter, E.M., Jones, A.M., Davison, R.R.C., Bromley, P.D. and Mercer, T.H. (eds.) (2006b). *The British Association of Sport and Exercise Sciences Sport and Exercise Physiology Testing Guidelines Volume 2: Exercise and Clinical Testing.* London: Routledge.

World Health Organization (1998). *Obesity: preventing and managing the global epidemic: Report of a WHO consultation on Obesity.* Geneva: World Health Organization.

Chapter 7

Training and conditioning

Introduction

All athletes participate in training and conditioning activities, taking up an enormous amount of their time. An elite athlete might train most days but amateur athletes can also dedicate most of their leisure time to training. For this reason training should be both purposeful and enjoyable. Well-planned and effective training and conditioning is associated with optimising performance. Conversely, poor training and conditioning is associated with a plateau in fitness or a decrease in performance resulting in potential physiological and psychological harm. For example, overtraining syndrome can happen, leading to an increased risk of injury.

The major aims of training and conditioning for a sports therapist are to:

- act as a prehabilitation measure to address an athlete's or team's weaknesses so that these do not become a major cause of injury (for example, in football, core stability and proprioception training may enable safer changes in direction without injury)

- ensure rehabilitation programmes are both effective and safe, and do not lead to an athlete relapsing in their rehabilitation or suffering further injury

- optimise performance to enable athletes to participate effectively and reach their full athletic potential

- optimise the fitness of non-athletes in order to maintain or improve health, and reduce the risk of chronic disease in which low levels of activity may be one of the contributing factors such as diabetes type 2, cardiovascular disease and depression.

Learning outcomes

After you have read this chapter you should be able to:

- define fitness and its components

- explain fitness requirements of sport and exercise

- explain training theory

- explain how to prepare for training

- describe training methods.

Starting block

A rugby union player has been referred to you in a late stage of his rehabilitation. The player's objective is now to get himself up to full match fitness so that he performs well and doesn't incur injury.

- Explain and justify the physiological and psychological demands of the sport to the player.

Defining fitness and its components

Fitness is difficult to define because being 'fit' means different things to different people. For example, it can mean being able to lead a fulfilling and independent life and maintaining an aesthetically pleasing body image, or it can mean participating in a chosen sport to the highest level. Most definitions of fitness relate to being able to meet the demands of the environment without excessive fatigue or disease. The environmental demands placed on an individual can be broadly classified as:

- physical – undertaking activities of everyday life, participation in exercise and sport

- mental – the emotional and cognitive demands of everyday life

- social – the demands of interacting with others, e.g. family, friends, colleagues, and perceptions of body image.

Fitness has a close relationship with a number of other related terms such as **health**, well-being and quality of life. Having good levels of fitness is associated with maintaining positive physical, mental and social health. Poor levels of fitness are associated with poor physical and mental health and low levels of social interaction together with a threat to an individual's autonomy and independence (Paffenbarger, Lee, and Leung, 1994).

Health-related and performance-related fitness

Fitness can be divided into health-related fitness and performance-related fitness.

Health-related fitness is focused on areas that affect overall health and your ability to perform daily tasks and everyday activities. It is directly associated with the prevention of physical and mental disease, good quality of life, maintaining an active lifestyle and keeping above the **disability threshold**.

Key terms

Health – the general condition of the body or mind, especially in terms of the presence or absence of illnesses, injuries or impairments

Disability threshold – a threshold that determines an individual's autonomy and independence

Performance-related fitness focuses on the ability to perform specific skills which are required by various activities and sports. This type of fitness has little to do with overall health status and is much more performance and sport specific.

Both health-related and performance-related fitness are made up of a number of attributes or components. Although there is very little crossover between both types of fitness, an individual's balance can be seen as a health-related component of fitness due to balance deteriorating with age and thus directly impacting on health by increasing the risk of falls in the elderly. All of the fitness components are transient which means they can be easily improved through training and conditioning or detrained if they are neglected. For example, when an athlete has to cease training due to injury or in the off-season when training load reduces.

Table 7.1: Definitions of health-related fitness components

Fitness component	Definition
Cardiorespiratory endurance	The ability of the cardiorespiratory system to remove waste products and deliver oxygen and nutrients to the muscles to enable prolonged activity.
Muscular endurance	The capability of the muscles to contract repeatedly without fatigue. It is muscle specific.
Muscular strength	The maximum force that can be exerted on an object in one contraction. It is muscle specific.
Flexibility	The range of movement around a joint. This is joint specific.
Body composition	The proportion of lean tissue, fat, water, and mineral in the body.
Neuromuscular relaxation	The ability of the nervous system to contract and consequently relax the muscles.
Musculoskeletal fitness	The ability of the connective tissues to withstand strain, and the bones to absorb nutrients.

Table 7.2: Definitions of performance-related fitness components

Fitness component	Definition
Speed	The ability of body to complete a task quickly.
Power	The ability to generate maximum force quickly. It is a product of speed and strength. Often displayed as being weight relative, e.g. weight/power ratio.
Reaction time	The ability of the nervous and muscular systems to respond to a stimulus.
Co-ordination	The ability to perform two or more tasks at once.
Balance	The ability to remain in a set position for a period of time.
Agility	The ability to change direction quickly and effectively.

The term 'total fitness' refers to having the highest possible level of all the health-related and performance-related components of fitness. It is debatable whether an athlete can ever achieve total fitness because achieving high levels of one component could be associated with a reduction in others (Godfrey and White, 2006). For example, gaining muscle strength is linked to a reduction in flexibility, cardiorespiratory endurance, and muscle endurance. Nevertheless, encouraging an athlete to aspire towards total fitness can be beneficial in terms of motivation and **adherence** to training.

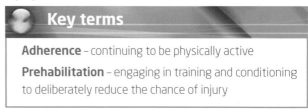

Stop and think

Which type of athletes do you think are close to achieving total fitness and why?

Fitness requirements of sport and exercise

When using training and conditioning for performance, **prehabilitation**, rehabilitation or health reasons, you must understand the fitness requirements of sport, exercise and lifestyle activity so that your client can be best conditioned to meet these requirements. If not, the individual will not be able to cope with the physical demand placed upon them and performance will decrease and the risk of injury increases.

Key terms

Adherence – continuing to be physically active

Prehabilitation – engaging in training and conditioning to deliberately reduce the chance of injury

Key fitness components

Each type of sport and exercise can be broken down into the key fitness components for which it requires high levels. These components should then be prioritised in a training or rehabilitation programme. For example, boxing requires high levels of agility, reaction time, muscle endurance and power – these components should be a priority when designing a training programme. Table 7.3 highlights the major fitness requirements of a range of individual and team sports.

Table 7.3: Essential fitness requirements of a range of sports

Sport	Essential fitness components
Marathon	Cardiorespiratory endurance, body composition, muscle endurance, flexibility
Triple jump	Power, balance, co-ordination, speed, flexibility
Basketball	Power, agility, cardiorespiratory endurance, muscle endurance, speed, balance
Rugby league	Cardiorespiratory endurance, power, muscle endurance, agility, speed, muscle strength
Swimming (50 m freestyle)	Reaction time, co-ordination, muscle endurance, speed, power

Activity

For the following sports and exercises rank each of the health- and performance-related fitness components out of 10 in terms of their importance.

Use a scale of 1 = unimportant, 10 = highly important and be able to justify your answers:
- 100 m sprinting
- 2000 m rowing
- Triathlon
- Gymnastics (floor performance).

Key training theory

If training and conditioning are to be effective, they must be directed and informed by theory. This allows individuals taking part in sport or exercise to perform at their best possible level and will facilitate continual improvement in their performance. Two training theories include the General Adaptation Syndrome (GAS: Selye, 1936) and the Supercompensation Cycle (Jakowlew, 1976).

General Adaptation Syndrome (GAS)

GAS has a number of stages that describe how the body reacts to training load and then how it responds to this.

1. The first stage is termed the 'shock' stage and refers to how the body responds to biological stress and tries to overcome the imbalance caused by this stress. In terms of training it is where the individual experiences soreness and tiredness caused by exercise.

2. The second or 'resistance' stage starts as soon as the stressor or exercise ceases and the body recovers from the temporary imbalance and adapts to a higher level of performance or fitness.

3. The third stage or the 'exhaustion' stage is reached when the body is overstressed for a long period of time and doesn't have enough time to adapt. Athletes who over train are the individuals who generally reach this stage. They may complain of staleness despite training hard.

Supercompensation Cycle

The Supercompensation Cycle is related to GAS and describes the link between training load and regeneration as the basis of improvements in fitness. This cycle has four parts:

- training
- fatigue
- recovery
- adaptations.

When an individual initially undertakes training it has a profound effect on the physiology of the body such as alteration to blood flow, changes in energy demand and build up of waste products. This accounts for temporary reductions in performance. Following this the body's **homeostasis** needs to be restored so that energy stores are replenished, waste products removed and micro trauma repaired. These functions occur in the recovery or compensation phase and only occur if adequate recovery is allowed. This recovery time is largely dependent on the intensity of the training and subsequent effect on the body's homeostasis. The third phase relates to **supercompensation** and how the body achieves a higher level of homeostasis. For example, more energy can be stored and there is greater aerobic or anaerobic ability.

Key terms

Homeostasis – the maintenance of a constant internal environment within the body

Supercompensation – positive adaptation made by the body following a period of training and recovery

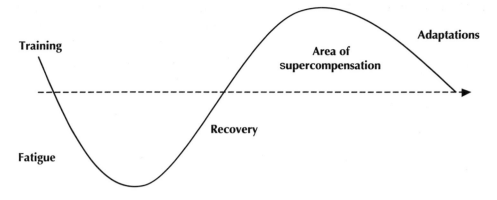

Figure 7.1: The supercompensation cycle applied to training and conditioning

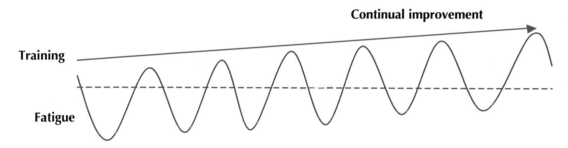

Figure 7.2: The chronic training model showing continual improvement over a period of time. How would this diagram change if insufficient recovery was allowed?

Over time, if enough recovery is allowed, an individual will undergo continual improvements in fitness as shown in Figure 7.2. If there is not enough recovery no improvements may occur or fitness/performance may decrease. Recovery is one of the most important components of a training programme. It repairs exercise induced tissue damage and allows tissues to adapt to improve fitness. Recovery can be active which involves reducing training load, having an 'easy' session, or changing to a different training method, e.g. swimming instead of running. Passive recovery is where an athlete would take part in very little or no activity and simply rest or receive sports massage.

Remember

A sports massage can be conducted as part of an athlete's recovery.

Specific Adaptation to Imposed Demand (SAID)

This explains that whatever demand is placed on the body it will adapt in a specific way (Godfrey and

Whyte, 2006). This is important when considering injury or performance. The type of contraction and speed, and intensity of training, will cause specific training effects. For example, training at submaximal levels develops slow twitch fibres, and in contrast high intensity will develop fast twitch anaerobic fibres. Any training should be specific to the physical demands of each sport. This entails considering the energy systems used, intensity, muscle group used, and components of fitness required. Specificity of function suggests that at an advanced stage of rehabilitation training should mirror the sport in order to mirror the intensity of competition, muscular demands and neural patterns of the sport (Godfrey and Whyte, 2006).

Progressive overload

This is essential in any training programme in order to continually improve fitness and avoid the fitness plateau. Fitness will improve as a result of training. However, the training stimulus (including frequency, duration and intensity) needs to be heightened in order for fitness to keep improving. Figure 7.2 represents how this would look if progressive overload is applied. For improvements in fitness and performance training work needs to be hard and to stress the body in order for successful adaptation to take place as Figure 7.1 demonstrates.

Reversibility

Reversibility in fitness occurs when the training stimulus is reduced or ceased. Generally the anaerobic ability of the body is lost before the aerobic ability. Reversibility may become evident as a result of injury or between competitive seasons. If reversibility occurs, care must be taken not to overstretch individuals and induce injury or **delayed onset of muscle soreness (DOMS)**.

Avoiding tedium

Training must include some variety in order to prevent it becoming a chore or tedious. Athletes spend a great deal of time training and it can often be exhaustive. It is important to change training methods and training goals, and mix up hard and easy sessions to avoid boredom.

Individual training needs

Every athlete who undergoes training and conditioning has their own unique individual genetics, medical background, fitness goals and fitness needs. Athletes of different ages and genders would need to be conditioned in different ways. For example, an athlete who is over 50 years old may need more recovery time, while maximal lifting is thought to be risky with under 16-year-olds.

Training phases and cycles

Many athletes train and compete throughout a season. Usually a season has a number of phases.

- Preparation phase – where basic general fitness is developed and restored through conditioning and where more sports specific fitness and techniques are developed in order to prepare for the intensity of competition.

- Competition phase – where athletes try to combine maintaining fitness over a period of time, competing and recovery.

- Transition phase – where there is a period of regeneration and recovery following a competitive season and training load is significantly decreased and there is no competition.

Throughout the season athletes need to achieve peak performance and fitness at the right time. Training programmes should be periodised so that long-term fitness goals can be broken down into shorter term aims. To achieve this, training programmes include macrocycles, mesocycles, and microcycles.

- The macrocycle is usually a long-term goal covering a full season or can be a four year goal for an Olympic athlete.

- A mesocycle is a medium-term goal and would cover preparation, transition and competition phases of a season.

- A microcycle is made up of short-term goals on a weekly or monthly basis and is part of a logical approach to how the macrocycle can be achieved through training and conditioning.

Key terms

Delayed Onset of Muscle Soreness (DOMS) – pain and stiffness felt in muscles several hours to days after unaccustomed and/or strenuous exercise. Delayed onset muscle soreness begins 8–24 hours after exercise and peaks 24–72 hours after exercise (Marcora and Bosio, 2007)

Periodisation – the purposeful variation of a training programme over time, so an athlete achieves peak performance prior to an event or competition

Not all athletes have the same competition calendar so there are different types of **periodisation**.

- Mono-cycle periodisation is where an athlete needs to peak for one competition during the season.

- Bi-cycle periodisation is peaking twice throughout a season.

- Tri-cycle periodisation is peaking for three competitions.

Preparing for training

When planning or conducting training and conditioning activities you need to prepare both the environment and the athletes to make training safer and more effective.

Risk assessments

A thorough risk assessment should be conducted of all training environments. For example, training outside on a sports field presents different risks and hazards from those of a strength and conditioning area in a gym. Table 7.4 highlights common hazards of indoor, outdoor and aqua environments.

A risk assessment will identify possible **hazards** and **risks** to the athlete and how these can be prevented or eliminated to provide a safe and effective environment.

Table 7.4: Common hazards in training and conditioning environments

Gym based	Outdoors	Aqua
• Tripping • Faulty equipment • Poor technique • Overexertion • Electrical equipment	• Poor technique • Weather (hot or cold) • Surface (e.g. frozen, hard, cambered) • Road traffic • Poor visibility	• Slipping • Drowning • Overexertion • Poor hygiene

Hazard	Risk	Severity of risk			Preventative measures
		Likelihood of risk (1-10)	Severity of risk (1-10)	Overall risk (high/ medium/low)	

Figure 7.3: An examplar template of a risk assessment

Activity

Using the template in Figure 7.3 conduct a risk assessment of your training and conditioning environment.

Medical screening

Review the medical screening of every client before any training. This will inform you about the readiness of the athlete to take part in training activities. You need to be aware of any medical contraindications to training and any medication that your client is taking so you can ensure that training is not potentially harmful to their health. This will inform the training programme you devise as certain activities may have to be avoided based on medical information. For example, for some athletes with exercise-induced asthma, sudden increases in intensity should be avoided to reduce the risk of an associated attack; hypertensive athletes should avoid **isometric** muscle conditioning work as this can cause a rapid rise in blood pressure.

Key terms

Hazard – a situation or object that could cause an accident or injury. For example, water on the floor is a hazard as it could cause someone to slip and fall

Risk – a risk is the likelihood that an accident might occur. For example, how likely is it that someone might slip on the water that has been spilled on the floor?

Isometric – where the muscle contracts without movement or is static

You may find it useful as part of medical screening to gain a holistic view of each athlete's lifestyle. Include stress, social support, previous exercise history, alcohol intake, smoking and diet in the factors you consider. Diet can have a major effect on training adaptations and athletic performance so ask questions about carbohydrate, protein and fluid intake, and any supplementation.

Fitness testing

A fitness appraisal of each athlete using fitness testing is essential prior to training and conditioning. This will inform you of each athlete's individual strengths and weaknesses so that they can be addressed. An athlete who is not fit enough to compete in their sport is likely to perform poorly and be at greater risk of sports injury.

Fitness testing may also be used to assess overall team or squad strengths and weaknesses. For example, poor team performance towards the end of games could be the result of fitness flaws. Effective and informed training goals can then be designed for the athlete or team using the correct SMARTS theory of goal setting. (See *Chapter 11: Psychology of sports injury* for more detail on the process of goal setting.)

Fitness testing can also be used to evaluate training and conditioning goals, and to identify signs of exhaustion and overtraining. For further information on the aims of fitness testing, and selecting and conducting appropriate tests, see *Chapter 6: Fitness testing for sports therapy*.

 Remember

Allow the athlete to take responsibility for creating fitness goals as this will increase their feelings of control and autonomy. It will also encourage them to stick to their training schedule.

Training methods

Training and conditioning should mimic the sport or exercise the athlete is training for as closely as possible. Selecting the wrong training method will reduce any training effect and ill prepare the athlete, leaving them at greater risk of fatigue and injury. For example, if an athlete's sport requires them to use a number of different energy systems and muscle fibre types, then the training method selected should develop this ability.

Most training methods can take place individually or in groups, and across a number of different environments such as indoor, outdoor and aqua. Table 7.5 identifies a range of training methods aimed at improving fitness, performance and rehabilitation.

The key elements of fitness that different training methods might be employed to develop are:

- cardiorespiratory endurance
- muscle conditioning including endurance, strength and power
- balance and stability

- speed, agility and quickness
- flexibility.

Table 7.5: Appropriate training methods to improve performance and facilitate rehabilitation

Key element	Training methods
Cardiorespiratory endurance	Long slow duration (LSD) training Threshold training Interval training Fartlek training
Muscle conditioning (strength, endurance, power)	Resistance training Plyometric training
Balance and stability	Core stability training Proprioception training
Speed, agility and quickness	Assisted sprint training Resisted sprint training Repetitive sprint training Speed, agility and quickness (SAQ) drills
Flexibility	Static stretching (active and passive) Dynamic stretching Proprioceptive neuromuscular facilitation (PNF)

 Remember

Before any training session, always include a good warm-up (including mobility, pulse raiser and stretching) and a cool-down including pulse decreaser and stretching.

Cardiorespiratory endurance

This can be developed by using training methods that differ by the intensity and duration of the activity (Londeree, 1997).

- **Long slow duration training** – focused on training at a fixed moderate intensity for a time period typically of between 60–120 minutes. This type of training tends to make up the majority of training time in endurance athletes.

- **Threshold training** – usually conducted over a moderate duration (30–60 minutes) at an intensity performed around the athlete's **lactate threshold** usually at 75–85 per cent of the athlete's maximum heart rate.

- **Interval training** – typically short duration and very high intensity. It is a structured training method involving repetitions of high intensity followed by a period of active recovery at a lower intensity. Usually the intense periods are above the athlete's lactate threshold. The duration and frequency of both the repetition and recovery periods can be adapted based on the athlete's needs.

- **Fartlek training** – tends to be unstructured and works an athlete across a range of intensities for a long duration. Walking, jogging, running and sprinting are all options in this training method. In the purest sense Fartlek training should take place over different terrains and tends to add variety to an athlete's training as no two sessions are the same.

Stop and think

Consider the demands of competing in football. Which training method is best suited to improve cardiorespiratory endurance?

Muscle conditioning

For muscle conditioning, resistance and plyometric training are common training methods.

- **Resistance training** is an umbrella term covering the use of free weights, body resistance, resistance machines, therabands and resistance provided in water. Depending on the athlete, resistance training can be used to isolate specific muscle groups or involve gross compound multi joint movements for performance and rehabilitation. To develop muscle endurance, the focus of resistance training is to apply moderate load for a large number of repetitions. For strength and muscle size, the focus should be on a near maximal load for very few repetitions. The amount of sets of this exercise and recovery can then differ. Care must be taken with resistance training to promote good technique when lifting near maximal load.

- **Plyometric training** is an established training method aimed at improving muscle power. This type of training involves fast, explosive movements aimed at improving the neuromuscular functioning and increasing

power from the **stretch shortening cycle (SSC)**. Repetitions of jumping and bounding exercises are typically used in plyometric training. As a result of the very high intensity of plyometric training, and subsequent stress on the body tissue, muscle soreness is common. Table 7.6 identifies plyometric exercise for the upper and lower body.

Table 7.6: A range of plyometric exercises for the lower and upper body

Lower body plyometric exercises	Upper body plyometric exercises
Squat jumps	Overhead throw
Jump to box	Side throw
Lateral jump to box	Over back toss
Single leg hop	Slams
Double leg hop	Explosive start throws
Split squat jump	Single arm overhead throw
Tuck jump	Squat throws
Lateral box push off	Plyometric push-up
Bounding	
Bounding with rings	
Box drills	
Lateral hurdle	
Depth jump	

Balance and stability

Improving balance and stability involves training both the muscles and the nerve receptors that determine proprioceptive ability. Core stability training includes any exercise that works the superficial and deep muscles of the trunk. Typical core stability exercises include the muscle movements of flexion, extension, rotation and lateral flexion. Repetitions of these exercises can be conducted on a mat, standing or on an uneven surface such as a core ball.

Key terms

Lactate threshold – the intensity of exercise where there is sustained increase in blood lactate above baseline values

Stretch shortening cycle (SSC) – defined as an active stretch (eccentric contraction) of a muscle followed by an immediate shortening (concentric contraction) of that same muscle and determined by elastic potential of muscles and nervous innervation

The main aim of **proprioception** training is to stress the nerve receptors that give joints their stability and balance in order to develop their ability. Exercises on wobble boards, standing on one leg, trampoline or any uneven surface will develop proprioceptive ability.

Speed, agility and quickness (SAQ)

In most sports, developing speed, agility and quickness is vital. Assisted or resisted sprints can be used in training to allow the athlete to sprint either with or against a force. An example of assisted sprinting would be sprinting downhill while an example of resisted sprinting would be running uphill, using a viper belt to provide resistance, or running with a parachute behind.

Assisted sprinting develops stride length and **cadence** while resisted sprints develop speed endurance. Repetition sprints in their basic form are repetitions of maximal sprints over a set distance with a structured rest period. SAQ drills include practising starting positions for sprinting, techniques of multi direction movement, changing direction effectively and promoting quick foot work. The use of hurdles, ladders, hoops and balls can make SAQ drills more sport specific.

Key terms

Proprioception – the body's ability to sense its positioning in open space and to determine the body's balance and stability

Cadence – the speed it takes to go through a full gait cycle

Flexibility

Developing flexibility is associated with more efficient sporting techniques, better force generation and reduction in injury.

Static stretching involves holding a muscle under strain for a set period of time. These stretches can be performed actively by the athlete or passively by the sports therapist. You should not stretch the muscle statically in a warm-up for more than 10 seconds as this can reduce muscle performance and increase risk of injury (Shrier, 2004).

Dynamic stretching involves the athlete stretching the muscle while moving. For example, the hamstrings can be stretched by mimicking kicking a ball. It is ideally suited to warming up as the stretches mimic sporting movements and do not reduce heart rate while performing them (as static stretching does).

Proprioceptive neuromuscular facilitation (PNF) (Knott and Voss, 1977) develops flexibility by placing a specific muscle in a forced isometric contraction to reduce how the nervous system and muscle fibres inhibit flexibility (Spernoga et al. 2001). Figure 7.4 illustrates the use of PNF to develop flexibility in the hamstrings.

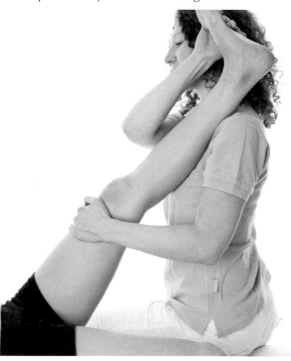

Figure 7.4: The use of PNF on the hamstring group. Typically the forced isometric contraction is held for 5–10 seconds then placed in a relaxed position before being held in a stretched position. This can then be repeated. What questions would you ask an athlete when performing PNF stretching to make sure it is safe and effective?

Remember

In a warm-up, stretches are generally held for 8–10 seconds and in a cool-down they are held for upwards of 15–30 seconds.

Case study

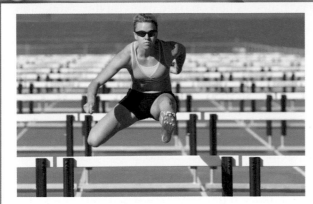

A heptathlete takes part in seven different events over 2 days. The events she competes in are 100 m hurdles, high jump, shot put, 200 m, long jump, javelin throw and 800 m. Such a variety of events has huge physiological demands on the athlete's body so her training and conditioning must prepare her body for this challenge. She is currently getting ready for her next major athletic event. Can you give her some training and conditioning advice?

1. What are the physiological demands of being a heptathlete?

2. Is it possible to be best in all seven events?

3. How can you ensure the athlete is at peak level performance around the time of the World Championships?

4. What would be the macro, meso and microcycles involved in a training programme for the athlete?

5. Which training methods would you use with this athlete and why?

Check your understanding

1. Why is the term fitness hard to define?

2. Name all of the health-related fitness components.

3. Name all of the performance-related fitness components.

4. Explain the supercompensation cycle.

5. Why is recovery important in training and conditioning?

6. Why is a fitness appraisal important in preparing for training and conditioning?

7. Explain the different phases in an athlete's competitive season.

8. Describe threshold training.

9. In general how can muscle strength and size be developed?

10. Describe the process of PNF stretching.

To obtain answers to these questions visit the companion website at www.pearsonfe.co.uk/foundationsinsport

Useful resources:

To obtain a secure link to the websites below, see the Websites section on page ii or visit the companion website at www.pearsonfe.co.uk/foundationsinsport.

Peak Performance Online

UK Strength and Conditioning Association

British Association of Sport and Exercise Sciences

Further reading

American College of Sports Medicine (2006). *ACSM's Guidelines for Exercise Testing and Prescription* 7th Edition. Philadelphia: Lippincott, Williams & Wilkins.

Cartwright, L.A. and Pitney, W.A. (2005). *Fundamentals of Athletic Conditioning* 2nd Edition. Champaign: Human Kinetics.

Chandler, J.T. and Brown, L.E. (2006). *Conditioning for Strength and Human Performance*. Philadelphia: Lippincott, Williams & Wilkins.

Dick, F.W. (2007). *Sports Training Principles* 5th Edition. London: A&C Black Publishers Ltd.

Foran, B. (2000). *High Performance Sports Conditioning*. Champaign: Human Kinetics.

French, D. (2008). *Conditioning the hamstrings: Training considerations for performance and injury prevention*, Vol.15, 18–22. sportEX Dynamics.

Godfrey, R., and Whyte, G., (2006) Training specificity. *In* Whyte, G., (2006) *The Physiology of Training: Advances in Sport and Exercise Science Series*. Philadelphia: Churchill Livingstone, Elsevier.

Hoff, J., Wisloff, U., Engen, L.C., Kemi, O.J. and Helgerud, J. (2002). Soccer specific aerobic endurance training. *British Journal of Sports Medicine*. Vol. 36(3), 218–222.

Jakowlew, N.N. (1977). *Sportbiochemie*. Leipzig: Barth

Knott, M., Viss, I., Myers, J.W. and Voss, D., (1985) *Proprioceptive Neuromuscular Facilitation*. Revised 3rd Edition. Philadelphia: Lippincott, Williams & Wilkins

Kreider, R.B., Fry, A.C. and O'Toole, M.L. (1998). *Overtraining in Sport*. Champaign: Human Kinetics.

Londeree, B.R., (1997) Effect of training on lactate/ventilator thresholds: a meta-analysis. *Medicine and Science in Sport and Exercise*. Vol. 29(6), 837–843

Marcora, S.M., and Bosio, A., (2007) Effect of exercise-induced muscle damage on endurance running performance in humans. *Scand J Med Science Sports*. Vol. 17, 662–671

Paffenbarger, R.S., Lee, I.M., & Leung, R. (1994) Physical activity and personal characteristics associated with depression and suicide in American college men. *Acta Psychiatrica Scandinavia*, Vol. 89, 16–22

Reilly, T. (2007). *The Science of Training – Soccer*. London: Taylor and Francis.

Selye, H. (1950) Stress and the General Adaptation Syndrome. *British Medical Journal*. Vol. 1, 1383

Shrier, I., (2004) Does stretching improve performance? A systematic and critical review of the literature. *Clinical Journal of Sports Medicine*. Vol. 14(5), 267–273

Spernoga, S.G., Uhl, T.L., Arnold, B.L., and Gansneder, B.M., (2001) Duration of Maintained Hamstring Flexibility After a One-Time, Modified Hold-Relax Stretching Protocol. *Journal of Athletic Training*. Vol. 36(1), 44-48

Whyte, G. (2006). *The Physiology of Training: Advances in Sport and Exercise Science Series*. Philadelphia: Churchill Livingstone, Elsevier.

Yakovlev, N. (1967) *Sports Biochemistry*. Leipzig. Deutsche Hochschule für Körperkultur

Chapter 8

Activity, nutrition and lifestyle management

Introduction

The nation's health is in a state of crisis and it is thought to be due to a lack of activity, poor dietary habits and poor lifestyle choices. Engaging in regular activity, eating a healthy diet, not smoking and sensible alcohol intake all have health improving qualities – alternatively, not doing so can have detrimental effects on health. A number of chronic diseases are related to the lifestyle management of activity, diet, smoking and alcohol including cardiovascular disease, diabetes type 2, obesity, osteoporosis, depression and cancer.

As well as affecting an individual's health, these diseases have huge social and economic consequences: they place a strain on the National Health Service (NHS) and lead to absenteeism in the workplace. An individual's decision to adhere to positive lifestyle choices is determined by personal, social and environmental factors. As a health care professional, you should understand exactly how lifestyle choices can affect health, the various factors determining lifestyle choices, and how an individual's behaviour can be changed for the better. It is only then that you can work holistically with your clients.

Learning outcomes

After you have read this chapter you should be able to:

- define physical activity, exercise and sport

- explain barriers to exercise participation

- explain the physical and psychological benefits of exercise

- explain the negative effects of exercise on health

- describe the components of a healthy diet

- explain how nutrition can improve sports performance and reduce risk of injury.

Definitions of physical activity, exercise and sport

If an individual chooses to become more active they face a number of options – whether to take part in more physical activity, exercise or sport, or a combination of all three. These terms are all different, though not mutually exclusive. You need to understand the subtle differences between them and how they relate to health and fitness. As a health care professional you must also understand why individuals do or do not engage in these different forms of activity.

● **Remember**

If you are conducting an activity-based research project, give a clear definition of the type/s of activity you will focus on and stick to it.

Physical activity is the movement of the body produced by skeletal muscles, resulting in increased energy expenditure and health improvements. Examples of physical activities include walking, housework, dancing, gardening and manual work. These are activities that make up 'normal' living. With greater reliance on technology to make life easier, and other leisure time alternatives such as playing computer games or watching television, levels of physical activity in the UK (such as walking and cycling) have dropped (Cutler, Glaeser, and Shapiro, 2003; Department of Health, 2004). Even a modest increase in physical activity can help maintain or improve health.

Exercise is a variation of physical activity. It is a planned, structured and repetitive activity that has a health-related or fitness-related objective. In crude terms it is physical activity with a fitness-based reason. Examples of exercise include gym training, circuit training jogging, and aerobics. Individuals participate in exercise for a number of reasons ssuch as:

● aesthetic (weight loss, muscle tone, etc.)

● gain/maintain health

● gain/maintain fitness

● stress relief

● social interaction.

Exercise is more positively related to health and fitness improvements than physical activity. However, exercise does have a number of negative effects on health such as addiction, eating disorders and injury which will be covered later in this chapter.

Sport is a variation of exercise. It is governed, rule bound and competitive, involving complicated movement patterns. Examples of sports include athletics, soccer, tennis, netball and basketball. Sport requires a greater level of skill and technique than other forms of activity. It also carries a much higher risk of injury when compared with physical activity and exercise.

All three activity types are conceptually based on an individual's reason for participation. For example, if an individual started cycling to work because it was less expensive than driving this would be physical activity. If the same individual decided to cycle at a weekend to lose weight this would be termed exercise. Finally, if this individual decided they were good at cycling and started to take part in road races this would be termed sport.

● **Stop and think**

There is a significant drop in activity levels in females aged 16 once they have left school. This is a concern as lifetime health is determined when you are younger. Why do you think this is the case?

Barriers to exercise participation

Taking part in recommended amounts of activity has a positive effect on an individual's health, while being **sedentary** is harmful to health. The recommended amount of activity to maintain health is:

- frequency – five or more times per week

- intensity – moderate intensity (55–70 per cent maximum heart rate)

- time – 30 minutes (continuous activity or accumulated throughout the day)

- type – cardiovascular-based activity (e.g. brisk walking, cycling, swimming, gardening, housework).

These activity guidelines could be met by engaging in physical activity, exercise, sport, or a combination of all three. The activity pyramid in Figure 8.1 demonstrates what a healthy active lifestyle should consist of with lots of **habitual physical activity** at the bottom and sedentary behaviour at the top.

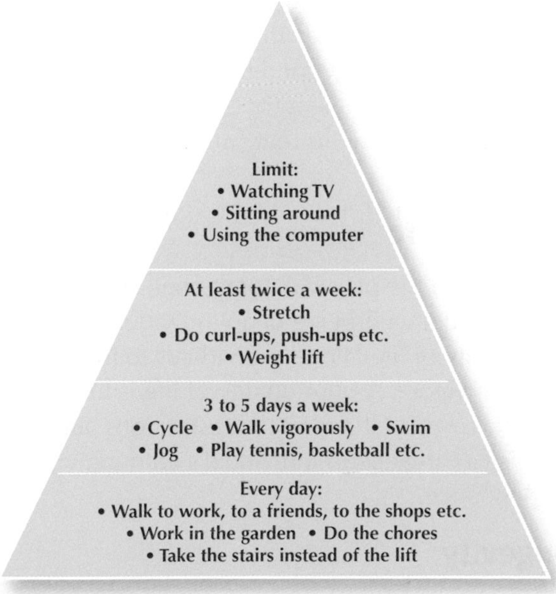

Figure 8.1: The activity pyramid for a healthy lifestyle

According to research conducted over the last few decades (Sports Council and Health Education Authority, 1992; **NHS Information Centre, 2008; Blair, 2009**) there is some agreement that:

- most individuals do not take part in enough activity to maintain health

- approximately a third of all adults are inactive (less than 30 minutes of activity per week)

- inactivity is more common than high blood pressure and smoking

- females take part in less activity than males

- worldwide inactivity accounts for a significant amount of disease burden and death

- the trend of inactivity extends to children.

There are international, regional and cultural variations in activity levels. For example, different regions in the UK report different activity levels depending on the socio-demographic make-up of the region (**NHS Information Centre, 2008**).

If you are to encourage clients to be more active for health, training and rehabilitation reasons, then understanding the common barriers to participation and key determinants of activity is important. The reasons why individuals do not take part in recommended activity levels is **multi-factorial**.

Key terms

Sedentary – a state of being physically inactive

Habitual physical activity – physical activity that is incorporated into everyday living

Multi-factorial – caused by many factors

Remember

If you are working with a client who you think won't stick to your training/rehabilitation plan, discuss the barriers they are worried about and how they can overcome them. This should help them stick to being active.

Table 8.1 identifies major perceived barriers to activity participation in adults.

Table 8.1: Common barriers to participation in adults

Barrier label	Barriers
Physical	I have an injury/disability that stops me. I'm too overweight. My health is not good enough. I'm too old.
Emotional	I'm not the 'sporty' type. I'm too shy or embarrassed. I might get injured or damage my health. I had a bad experience at school.
Motivational	I need to rest and relax in my spare time. I haven't got the energy after work. I'd never keep it up. I don't enjoy exercise.
Time	I haven't got the time. I don't have the time after work. I've got children to look after.
Availability	There is no one to do it with. I can't afford it. There are no suitable facilities nearby. I haven't got the right clothes or equipment.

(Sports Council and Health Education Authority, 1992)

Stop and think

As a sports therapist what advice would you give someone that uses the following barriers to participation?

- I have had a bad experience of sport and so I'm not the sporty type.
- I don't have the time to be active.
- My health isn't good enough.
- I've got children to look after.

Why do we participate?

You also need to explore what determines an individual's willingness to participate in activity. Human behaviour such as activity participation is determined by environmental, social, cognitive, physiological and personal factors.

Table 8.2: Key determinants of activity participation

Determinants	Examples
Environmental	Weather, media, air pollution, access to convenient facilities, personal safety, amount of leisure time
Social	Social modelling (in media and face to face), social support (friends, family, exercise professional)
Cognitive	Personal attitudes, beliefs, values, emotions, **self efficacy,** self concept and motivation
Physiological	Gender, health status, fitness status, fatigue resistance, ability
Personal	Exercise history, level of education, personal/family income, personality, social status

Key physical and psychological benefits of activity

Research suggests that being active has a protective effect on physical and mental health, and that it can be used to treat poor health (Blair et al., 1989; Dimeo, Bauer, Varaham, Proest, and Halter, 2001; Brosse, Sheets, Lett, and Blumenthal, 2002; Fogelholm, 2010). Doctors can now refer patients to exercise specialists if they think that activity could prevent or treat certain conditions. However, in order to maintain the benefits of activity, it must be regular. General benefits that can be gained include the following.

Quality of life

This relates to the physical, functional, social and emotional well-being of an individual. A good quality of life allows individuals to fulfil tasks with vigour. A poor quality of life is full of physical, emotional and social restrictions and becomes a threat to an individual's autonomy and independence.

Longevity

This relates to life expectancy. Leading an active lifestyle is associated with living a longer life as it slows the deterioration of a number of body systems. Leading an inactive or sedentary life is associated with a range of life threatening diseases and shorter life expectancy.

Disease prevention and treatment

Evidence suggests that engaging in regular activity can play an important role in the prevention of **chronic disease** and its treatment for those already diagnosed (Kokkinos, 2008; Faul et al., 2011). Figure 8.2 illustrates the chronic diseases that can be partly attributed to an inactive lifestyle. Many of these chronic diseases are interlinked. For example, an individual who suffers from obesity may suffer diabetes type 2 due to insulin resistance associated with excess body fat, and from high blood pressure caused by fatty deposits lining the blood vessels.

The precise mechanism behind why activity can help prevent and aid the treatment of specific chronic diseases is not entirely clear. It is thought that the true benefit of activity comes from

the interaction of physical and psychological mechanisms. Table 8.3 identifies key mechanisms that help with the prevention and treatment of specific chronic diseases. The psychological benefits of activity are important in improving the quality of life for all those suffering from chronic diseases as they may have lowered self-esteem, confidence and **self efficacy**.

Key terms

Chronic disease – diseases that an individual suffers with for months and years – they are long-lasting and recurrent

Self efficacy – the belief that an individual has in their own abilities to reach a specific goal or perform to a certain level

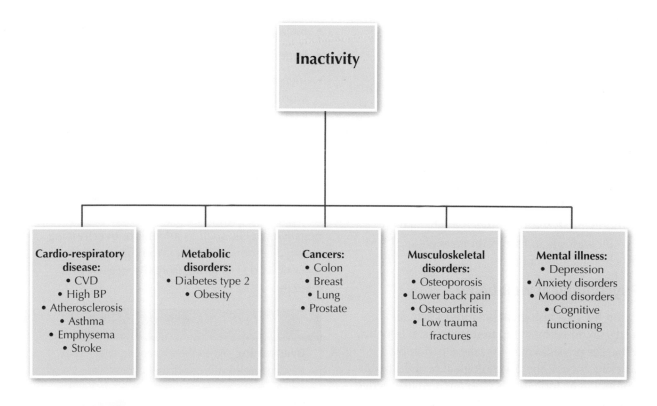

Figure 8.2: Health risks associated with leading an inactive lifestyle

Table 8.3: Key mechanisms behind the benefit of activity in the prevention and treatment of chronic disease

Cardiovascular disease	Obesity	Diabetes type 2	Osteoporosis	Depression
• Reduced BP • Reduced blood lipids • Less insulin resistance • Better blood vessel functioning • Reduced thrombosis risk • Psychological benefits	• Improved insulin sensitivity • Less insulin resistance • Increased metabolism • Improved energy balance • Reduction in body fat • Reduction in visceral fat • Psychological benefits	• Improved insulin sensitivity • Less insulin resistance • Better blood glucose control • Reduction in body fat • Psychological benefits	• Optimise peak bone mass • Maintain bone mineral density • Better posture • Reduction in body fat • Reduced joint deterioration • Improved balance, strength and co-ordination • Psychological benefits	• Improved sleep • Reduced muscle tension • Social interaction • Altered brain chemistry • Improved brain blood flow • Management of stress/anxiety • Better self-esteem/ self efficacy • Improved cognitive functioning

(adapted from Department of Health, 2004)

Weight management

Successful weight management means that an individual has a healthy weight. Being overweight and underweight is associated with the development of chronic disease and reduced life expectancy. Effective weight management is determined by both diet and activity. Specific dietary information will be covered later in the chapter. Increased amount of activity will increase metabolism and thus energy expenditure leading to a reduction or maintenance of weight. For individuals who are underweight, activity that increases lean tissue can have physical and psychological benefits.

Psychological well-being

Often the psychological benefits of activity are understated when compared to physical benefits. Whereas physical benefits take a period of weeks to occur, the psychological benefits occur immediately. Individuals who are regularly active report:

- increased positive mood states
- better stress management
- fewer incidents of mental illness

- feelings of vigour and energy
- better concentration
- increased confidence and perception of self-worth
- better body image.

Negative effects of exercise on health

Although there are huge health benefits in engaging in regular activity, there are also a number of negative effects, such as addiction, **overtraining**, eating disorders and injury. You may come across a client who is suffering from the negatives of exercise.

Key term

Overtraining – when the volume and intensity of training exceeds the body's ability to recover

Remember

If you suspect a client is suffering from an addiction or eating disorder it is in your duty of care to refer this individual. It is beyond a sports therapist's scope of practice.

There is a strong link between engaging in activity and eating disorders. The link is so strong that one of the diagnostic criteria for determining an eating disorder is excessive activity. Individuals who are suffering with an eating disorder may see activity as an added vehicle alongside dieting to aid excessive weight loss or see excessive activity as 'purging' themselves. The two eating disorders that this is particularly true of are **anorexia nervosa** and **bulimia nervosa**.

Key terms

Anorexia nervosa – an eating disorder associated with starvation of the body and excessive exercise

Bulimia nervosa – an eating disorder associated with bingeing on food/drink and then purging through not eating, excessive exercise or laxative use

There is some debate about whether individuals can become addicted to activity or whether this is another phenomenon such as an obsessive compulsive disorder. Research dating back decades has found that certain individuals do feel compelled and obliged to engage in excessive amounts of activity despite reporting no enjoyment (Morgan 1979; Szabo, 1995; Adams and Kirkby, 1997). These individuals are often associated with endurance-based exercise/sports.

Key negative behaviours that a sports therapist needs to be aware of in athletes include:

- being active despite being ill or injured
- excessive aimless activity without rest
- over concern with body weight/image
- maintaining a strict training/dietary regime
- becoming anxious, angry, guilty if training is missed
- structuring any social activity around being active.

Injury risk and overtraining are covered in *Chapter 2: Introduction to sports injury and assessment* and *Chapter 7: Training and conditioning.*

Components of a healthy diet

The effects of what we eat and drink on our health have become of increasing interest to the public. Nutrition and diet are two terms that are used extensively within society and the media.

- Nutrition refers to the science of feeding the body, or more specifically the sum of the processes of ingestion, digestion, assimilation and absorption of food and drink.

- Diet is a term that is commonly misused and often associated with restricting food and drink intake in some way. Essentially diet is best described as the food and drink you consume on a regular basis.

To understand what constitutes a healthy diet you must know which nutrients the body needs and the functions and sources of these nutrients. Like activity, a healthy diet is associated with good health and longevity, whereas an unhealthy diet is associated with poor quality of life, disease and premature death. A long-term poor diet can be a contributing factor to the progression of disease in the following:

- osteoporosis
- diabetes type 2
- irritable bowel syndrome (IBS)
- depression
- cardiovascular disease (CVD)
- stroke
- obesity
- high blood pressure and cholesterol
- cancer (bowel, colon, lung, breast, etc.)
- immune problems
- fatigue.

Remember

A client may ask you about nutrition and diet and you can give him or her dietary advice. However, manipulating an individual's diet is beyond a sports therapist's scope of practice.

Six essential nutrients

A healthy diet should be made up of a combination of essential nutrients. The six nutrients that are needed to maintain health are:

- carbohydrate (including fibre)
- fat
- protein
- water
- vitamins
- minerals.

Excessive intake or reduced intake of any of these key nutrients will lead to the body becoming malnourished and threatens health. Two basic examples of this are excessive vitamin C intake which is associated with dehydration, and excessive carbohydrate intake by an inactive individual which is associated with increases in body fat.

Macronutrients and micronutrients

- Macronutrients include carbohydrate, fat, protein and water and are required by the body in large quantities on a daily basis.
- Micronutrients include vitamins, minerals and trace elements and are needed in much smaller quantities.

Table 8.4: Examples of the major macronutrients and micronutrients

Macronutrients (>1g/day)	Micronutrients (<1g/day)
Carbohydrate (including fibre) Fat Protein Water	Vitamins Minerals Trace elements

Energy and energy balance

Humans need to eat and drink to provide the body with energy. The most common unit that is used on food labelling to describe how much energy it contains is the **kilocalorie (kcal)**. The more kilocalories in food and drink, then the more energy it contains.

A typically active male will require around 2500 kilocalories per day, while an active female will require 2000 kilocalories per day. The nutrients that provide the body with energy are:

- carbohydrate (4 kcals per gram)
- fat (8 kcals per gram)
- protein (4 kcals per gram)
- alcohol (7 kcals per gram).

The energy balance is the relationship between the amount of energy an individual takes in versus the amount of energy expended.

energy balance = energy intake – energy expenditure

The food and drink you consume typically makes up our energy intake. Energy expenditure is made up of the **thermic effect of activity**, **basal metabolic rate (BMR)**, and the **thermic effect of food**.

Key terms

Kilocalorie (kcal) – the amount of energy required to heat 1 litre of water by 1°C

Thermic effect of activity – the effect of activity on metabolic rate

Basal metabolic rate (BMR) – the amount of energy required to keep the body functioning at total rest

Thermic effect of food – the effect of food on metabolic rate

If an individual regularly has a positive energy balance they will typically gain weight. Alternatively if an individual regularly has a negative energy balance they will typically lose weight. This is the basic principle than underpins most modern diets.

Remember

One of the easiest ways to calculate your energy balance is to keep a daily food/drink and activity diary and calculate total energy intake versus expenditure. This will be even more reliable if it is done over a longer period of time.

Carbohydrate

The primary function of carbohydrate is to provide the body with energy. Traditionally carbohydrates were classified as simple (or sugars) and complex (or starches).

- Simple carbohydrates were associated with short-term energy release because of their simple chemical structure, e.g. glucose, sucrose.

- Complex carbohydrates such as glycogen and starch were associated with sustained energy release as a result of their more complex chemical structure.

Figure 8.3 shows the structures of simple and complex carbohydrates.

A better way to look at carbohydrates is by examining the **glycaemic index (GI)**. This is the rate of digestion and absorption of carbohydrate, ultimately affecting blood glucose levels.

- **High GI carbohydrates** – digested and absorbed relatively quickly. These are associated with a rapid rise in blood glucose followed by a rapid fall caused by the hormone insulin.

- **Low GI carbohydrates** – digested and absorbed more slowly, leading to a more sustained energy release without the excessive rise and fall seen with high GI carbohydrates.

- **Medium–low GI carbohydrates** – nutritionally, these are much better for health and quality of life.

Table 8.5 indentifies high, medium and low GI sources of carbohydrates.

Key terms

Glycaemic index (GI) – the rate of digestion and absorption of carbohydrate, or how quickly carbohydrate eaten raises blood glucose levels

Monosaccharide – a single sugar molecule. For example, glucose, fructose, galactose

Disaccharide – two monosaccharide molecules joined together. For example, sucrose is glucose and fructose bonded together

Polysaccharide – a large chain of monosaccharides. For example, glycogen is a huge chain of glucose molecules

---

monosaccharide (glucose)

disaccharide (sucrose)

polysaccharide (starch)

Figure 8.3: The chemical structure of simple (sugars) and complex carbohydrates (starches)

Table 8.5: Examples of high, medium and low GI sources of carbohydrate

High GI	Medium GI	Low GI
Boiled potato	Porridge	Honey
Sports drinks	Rice	Most fruit/fruit
Baked potato	Milk chocolate	juice
White bread	bars	Beans
Watermelon	Canned fruit	Lentils
Corn flakes	Cakes	Muesli
Bagel	Biscuits	Wholemeal bread
Sugar	Pastries	Wholemeal pasta/
Jam	Pasta	rice
Sweets		Nuts
Energy drinks		Vegetables
		Bran cereal

Protein

Protein is associated with the growth, repair and development of the body's tissues. The tissue types include: muscle, skin, hair, nails, organs, teeth, bones and connective tissue. Protein is also responsible for immune system function, production of hormones/**enzymes**, and is an important back-up source to meet energy needs in addition to carbohydrate and fat. Limited protein intake is associated with fatigue and poor immune function. Excessive protein is also harmful to health and is related to dehydration, mood swings and kidney damage.

Proteins are complicated structures made up of amino acids. Certain amino acids can be made by the body and are called non-essential amino acids. By comparison, essential amino acids cannot be made by the body so there is a need to obtain these through food and drink. Table 8.6 identifies the major essential and non-essential amino acids.

Table 8.6: Major essential and non-essential amino acids

Non-essential amino acids	Essential amino acids
Alanine	Histidine
Arginine	Isoleucine
Asparagine	Leucine
Aspartate	Lysine
Cysteine	Methionine
Glutamate	Phenylalanine
Glutamine	Threonine
Glycine	Trytophan
Proline	Valine
Serine	
Tyrosine	

- **Complete proteins** – are food sources that contain all the body's required essential amino acids. They come from mainly animal sources such as meat, fish and eggs.

- **Incomplete proteins** – are food sources that contain a limited number of essential amino acids. They come from vegetable sources such as nuts, pulses, seeds and grains.

Stop and think

Why might a vegetarian find it a challenge to get a healthy protein intake?

Fat

People immediately associate fat intake with the obesity epidemic (and indeed fats are a very rich energy source for the body). However, fats (and their smallest unit, fatty acids) are extremely important nutrients to maintain health; some fats are associated with preventing a number of chronic diseases.

The key function of fat is that it is a rich source of energy. You can store much more energy in your body in fat than carbohydrates. Fat cushions and protects vital organs, and is an important component in developing and repairing cell membranes. The production of a number of important hormones in the body relies on a healthy fat intake. Limited fat intake can restrict the production of these hormones.

Depending on their chemical structure, fats can be saturated or unsaturated.

- Saturated fats are solid at room temperature and tend to come from animal sources. High intake of these fats has been linked to a number of chronic diseases such as cardiovascular disease (CVD) and cancer. Trans-fats or man-made fats share similar characteristics to saturated fats and are also potentially harmful to health.

- Unsaturated fats are liquid at room temperature and tend to come from vegetable sources. Although high intake of unsaturated fats is not advisable, it is preferable to eat more unsaturated fats than saturated fats. Certain unsaturated fats such as **omega-3 fats** have been found to be beneficial to health by improving circulatory and mental health, and thus reducing the risk of CVD and depression.

Most sources of fat contain a mix of saturated and unsaturated fats. For example, butter contains mainly saturated fats, while vegetable oil contains mainly unsaturated fats.

Macronutrients

The proportion of macronutrients that an individual should consume on a daily basis can be seen in Figure 8.4.

Key terms

Enzymes – a type of protein with specific catalytic roles in metabolic reactions

Omega-3 fats – polyunsaturated fats that particularly come from oily fish and seed sources and have a positive effect on health

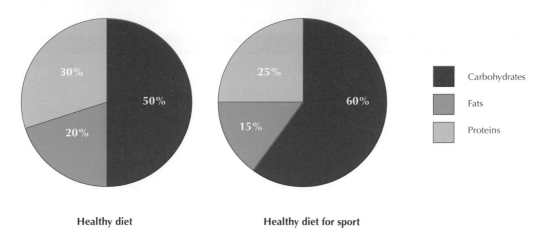

Carbohydrates	
Fats	
Proteins	

Healthy diet   Healthy diet for sport

Figure 8.4: The contribution of carbohydrate, fat and protein to overall energy intake in various groups

In this diagram the average diet relates to what the majority of the population consumes. A healthy diet gives guidelines on what is needed to maintain health. The sport diet reflects increased levels of activity to total energy; intake for sport will be much greater than the average or healthy diet.

Stop and think

What are the major differences in the two diagrams? What would happen if an inactive individual consumed a diet for sport?

Water

Water is the most abundant nutrient in the body accounting for around 65 per cent of body mass. It can be argued to be the most important nutrient. The body can withstand the effects of starvation for longer than it can withstand the effects of dehydration. Water has a range of functions such as:

* transporting key nutrients around and out of the body

* protecting through lubrication, cleaning and cushioning

* regulating body temperature

* acting as a solvent so substances can be dissolved into solutions.

The body gains and loses water in a number of ways as Table 8.7 identifies.

Table 8.7: Major mechanisms of water loss and gain on a daily basis

Water losses per day	Water gains per day
Sweat – water for cooling Excretion – water in urine and faeces Gaseous exchange – water vapour in expired air Diffusion – evaporative losses	Water in food and drink Metabolic – water resulting from breaking down of energy sources

Stop and think

Using Table 8.7, what is the rationale behind:
* drinking more on a hot day

* not exercising after suffering a recent episode of diarrhoea

* drinking more during activity?

Micronutrients

While micronutrients, including vitamins and minerals, are needed in much smaller quantities than macronutrients, they still have an important role to play in maintaining health.

Table 8.8: The function and sources of the major vitamins

Vitamin	Food sources	Major functions
Vitamin C	Green leafy vegetables, brightly coloured vegetables, citrus fruit, berries, tomatoes	Maintains connective tissue, cartilage, and bone. Helps with iron absorption, wound healing, protects against free radicals
Vitamin B1 (Thiamine)	Meat, yeast, wholegrain products, nuts, all vegetables	Energy production through carbohydrate. Nerve and heart function
Vitamin B2 (Riboflavin)	Milk and milk products, yeast, eggs, wholegrain products, green leafy vegetables	Cofactor in energy release
Niacin	Meat, liver, fish, eggs, yeast, wholegrains, peanuts	Energy release from carbohydrate and fat
Vitamin B6	Meat, wholegrain products, yeast, cereal products, peanuts, bananas, vegetables	Role in energy release from protein and carbohydrate
Vitamin B12	Liver, meat, dairy products, sardines, oysters, yeast extract	Formation of genetic material. Development of red blood cells
Folic acid	Liver, meat, fish, green leafy vegetables, orange juice	Formation of genetic materials, maintenance of red blood cells, involved in amino acid production
Vitamin A	Liver, dairy foods, green leafy vegetables, fruits	Essential for normal growth and development. Prevents night blindness. Maintenance of skin and surface cells
Vitamin D	Eggs, butter, liver, fish oils, fortified foods	Growth and development of bone. Helps with calcium and phosphorus absorption
Vitamin E	Vegetable oils, nuts, seeds, wholegrain products, green leafy vegetables, wheatgerm	Red blood cell production. As an antioxidant protects cell membranes and destroys free radicals
Vitamin K	Liver, meat, green leafy vegetables, soya beans, cabbage, cauliflower	Blood clotting, facilitates bone and kidney proteins

In Table 8.8 water soluble vitamins are not shaded, whereas fat soluble vitamins are shaded. Typically, excessive amounts of water soluble vitamins will have a diuretic action on the body; excessive fat soluble vitamins intake can be more harmful as these can be stored. In Table 8.9 the macrominerals (which the body needs in larger amounts) are shaded; microminerals are needed in much smaller quantities.

Table 8.9: The function and sources of major minerals

Mineral	Food sources	Major functions
Calcium	Milk, cheese, diary products, green leafy vegetables, canned fish, sesame seeds	Bone structure, blood clotting, nerve transmission, muscle contraction
Chlorine	Common table salt	Maintains electrolyte and fluid balance
Magnesium	Wholegrain products, green leafy vegetables, fruits, most other vegetables	Involved in regulation of protein synthesis, muscle contraction, temperature regulation, energy production
Phosphorus	Milk, poultry, fish, meat	Formation of blood and teeth, essential for normal use of B vitamins
Potassium	Meat, fish, poultry, cereals, bananas, milk, vegetables	Muscle function, nerve transmission, maintenance of body fluid balance
Sodium	Table salt, soy sauce, shellfish, yeast extract, canned meat	Has an important co-role with potassium to carry out body fluid balance
Iron	Liver, red meat, dried apricots, spinach, kidney beans, green leafy vegetables	Essential for red blood cell function and transport of oxygen
Copper	Meat, vegetables, fish, oysters, common in tap water	Components of many enzymes, aids function of red blood cells
Fluoride	Added to tap water, tea, fish	Prevents tooth decay, potential role in prevention of osteoporosis
Selenium	Meat, fish, wholegrain products	As an antioxidant destroys free radicals and protects cells from oxidative damage
Zinc	Meat, eggs, liver, oysters, wholegrain products, legumes	Component of many enzymes, aids wound healing, factor in protein and carbohydrate usage

Stop and think

Which of the vitamins and minerals above could be key to preventing sports injuries? What advice could you give a client to help them to increase their vitamin and mineral intake?

Nutrition to improve sports performance and reduce the risk of injury

At every level of sport it is extremely common for individuals to supplement their diet in order to improve performance, train harder, and recover quicker. In a study by Bayliss, Cameron-Smith, and Burke (2001) found that out of 77 elite swimmers 99 per cent reported supplementing their diets. The key problems with athletic supplements are (Burke and Deakin, 2006):

- the regulation of supplements in relation to ingredients and claims – as this industry has little regulation

- actual benefits – these are often claims and not supported by scientific findings

- side effects – some supplements may have adverse side effects

- supplements can foster a 'short cut' mentality and detract from actual priorities

- doping outcomes – some may contain ingredients banned by doping agencies. See the UK Anti-doping and the Global Drug Reference Online websites for more information on this.

What an active individual eats and drinks can affect both their personal performance and determine the risk of sport injury. Table 8.10 explains the role of key nutritional factors.

Table 8.10: Nutritional factors that can improve performance and reduce the risk of injury

Nutritional factor	Effect on performance and injury risk
Additional carbohydrate intake via food, fluid, or gels	Ensure carbohydrate stores are full before performance – vital for stamina and to delay fatigue Fatigued muscles cannot withstand the demands of performance and could sustain injury Low levels of carbohydrate are associated with poor concentration and poor decision making, increasing the risk of injury There is a need for additional carbohydrate intake before, during, and after performance
Maintaining hydration status	Good hydration delays fatigue caused by overheating and use of energy stores An individual suffering with dehydration will perform less well, overheat, appear confused/irritable and ultimately suffer cardiovascular collapse Certain supplements such as glycerol claim to allow individuals to hyperhydrate
Increased protein intake (amino acids)	Associated with better training adaptations and reduced fatigue Limited protein can lead to overtraining, immune problems and muscle soreness Certain supplemented proteins such as branched chained amino acids claim to reduce central fatigue
Intake of antioxidants	Activity produces a number of harmful substances called free radicals. These can cause muscle soreness and immune problems. Intake of antioxidants such as vitamins C, E and selenium destroy free radicals and can preserve health.
Use of nutritional supplements	Active individuals regularly take nutritional supplements to improve performance, e.g. caffeine, and creatine to recover from training e.g. glutamine and hydroxymethlybutrate (HMB), and to prevent injury, e.g. glucosamine and chondroitin

Case study

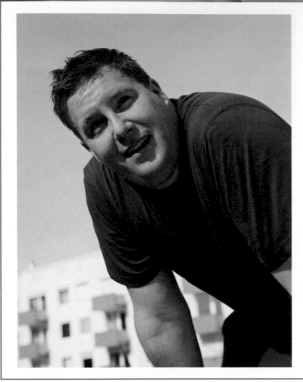

John is 34 years old, overweight, and describes himself as a 'slug'. He stopped taking part in exercise at the age of 16 years when it was no longer compulsory. In a recent doctor's appointment he was found to have moderately high blood pressure and that an additional weight gain could increase his chance of diabetes type 2. This has given John extra motivation to be more active and he has challenged himself to complete a 10 kilometre race for charity. He has not been to see anyone for advice on preparing himself for this and simply is going out for a run 6 times a week.

1. What might have led to John not maintaining an active lifestyle after school?

2. What psychological and physical health benefits might he gain from this challenge?

3. What are the potential health risks of undertaking this challenge?

4. What nutritional advice could you offer to improve his performance and to reduce his risk of injury?

Check your understanding

1. What are the key differences between physical activity, exercise and sport?

2. Why do individuals usually engage in activity?

3. Name five barriers to engaging in activity.

4. What is the recommended amount of activity that individuals should take part in to maintain health?

5. Describe the mechanisms relating to how activity can benefit osteoporosis.

6. Name five psychological benefits of activity.

7. What are the six essential nutrients that make up a healthy diet?

8. What is the glycaemic index?

9. What is the major difference between micronutrients and macronutrients?

10. Explain the energy balance and how this affects weight.

To obtain answers to these questions visit the companion website at www.pearsonfe.co.uk/foundationsinsport

Useful resources

To obtain a secure link to the websites below, see the Websites section on page ii or visit the companion website at www.pearsonfe.co.uk/foundationsinsport.

SportEx

World Health Organization

Medinfo for patients

Health Development Agency (formerly HEA), part of NICE

NHS Information Centre

American College of Sports Medicine

British Heart Foundation Statistics

National Institute for Health and Clinical Excellence

British Nutrition Foundation

Gatorade Sports Science Institute

Further reading

Adams, J., and Kirkby, R. (1997) Exercise Dependence: A Problem for Sports Physiotherapists. *Australian Journal of Physiotherapy*. Vol. 43(1), 53–58.

Allender, S., Scarborough, P., Peto, V., Rayner, M., Leal, J., Luengo-Fernandez and R., Gray, A. (2008). *European CVD statistics*. Brussels: European Heart Network.

ACSM (2005). *ACSM's Guidelines for Exercise Testing and Prescription* 2nd Edition. Philadelphia: Lippincott, Williams & Wilkins.

Bayliss, A., Cameron-Smith, D., and Burke, L.M., (2001) Inadvertent Doping Through Supplement Use by Athletes; Assessment and Management of Risk in Australia. *International Journal of Sports Nutrition and Exercise Metabolism*. Vol. 11, 365–383.

Biddle, S.J.H. and Mutrie, N. (2001, 2007). *Psychology of Physical Activity: Determinants, Well-being and Interventions*. London: Routledge.

Blair, S.N., Kohl, H.W., Paffenbarger, R.S., Clark, D.G., Cooper, K.H., and Gibbons, L.W. (1989) Physical fitness and all-cause mortality: a prospective study of healthy and unhealthy men. *Journal of the American Medical Association*. Vol. 262, 2395–2401.

Blair, S.N. (2009) Physical inactivity: the biggest public health problem of the 21st century. *British Journal of Sports Medicine*. Vol. 43, 1–2.

Brosse, A.L., Sheets, E.S., Lett, H.S., Blumenthal, J.A (2002) Exercise and the treatment of clinical depression in adults: Recent findings and future directions. *Sports Medicine*. Vol. 32(12), 741–760.

Buckworth, J. and Dishman, R.K. (2002). *Exercise Psychology*. Champaign: Human Kinetics.

Burke, L., and Deakin, V. (2006) *Clinical Sports Nutrition*, 3rd Edition. Sydney: McGraw-Hill

Camacho, T.C., Roberts, R.E., Lazarus, N.B., Kaplan, G.A. and Cohen, R.D. (1991). Physical activity and depression: Evidence from the Alameda county study. *American Journal of Epidemiology*, Vol. 134, 220–231.

Cutler, D. M., Glaeser, E. L. and Shapiro, J. M. (2003) Why Have Americans Become More Obese? *Journal of Economic Perspectives*, Vol. 17(3), 93-118.

Department of Health (2004) *At least five times a week: Evidence on the impact of physical activity and its relationship to health*. London: Department of Health. Available from http://www.dh.gov.uk

Department of Health (2008). *Health Survey of England 2006*. London: Department of Health.

Dimeo, F., Bauer, M., Varaham, I., Proest, G., Halter, U. (2001) Benefits from aerobic exercise in patients with major depression: a pilot study. *British Journal of Sports Medicine*, Vol. 35(2), 114.

Faul, L.A, Jim, H.S., Minton, S., Fishman, M., Tanvetyanon, T., and Jacobsen, P.B., (2011) Relationship of Exercise to Quality of Life in Cancer Patients Beginning Chemotherapy. *Journal of Pain Symptom Management*. Vol. 41(5), 859–69.

Fogelholm, M., (2010) Physical activity, fitness and fatness: relations to mortality, morbidity and disease risk factors. A systematic review. *Obesity Review*. Vol. 11, 202–21.

Griffin, J.C. (1998). *Client Centred Exercise Prescription*. Champaign: Human Kinetics.

Hardman, A.E. and Stensel, D.J. (2003). *Physical Activity and Health: The Evidence Explained*. London: Routledge.

Jackson, A.W., Morrow, J.R., Hill, D.W. and Dishman, R.K. (2004). *Physical Activity for Health and Fitness*. Champaign: Human Kinetics.

Jeukendrup, A. and Gleeson, M. (2004). *Sport Nutrition: An Introduction to Energy Production and Performance*. Champaign: Human Kinetics.

Kokkinos, P. (2008) Physical Activity and Cardiovascular Disease Prevention: Current Recommendations. *Angiology*. Vol. 59, 26–29.

Morgan, W.P., (1979) Negative Addiction in Runners. *The Physician and Sports Medicine*. Vol. 7, 57–63.

NHS Information Centre (2008) Health Survey for England 2008: Physical Activity and Fitness. Available from www.ic.nhs.uk.

NHS Information Centre (2008) Statistics on Obesity, Physical Activity, and Diet, England, January 2008. Available from www.ic.nhs.uk

Organisation for Economic Co-operation and Development (2010) Obesity and the Economics of Prevention: Fit not Fat - United Kingdom (England) Key Facts. Available from www.oecd.org/health/fitnotfat

Paffenbarger, R.S., Lee, I.M. and Leung, R. (1994). Physical activity and personal characteristics associated with depression and suicide in American college men. *Acta Psychiatrica Scandinavia*, Vol. 89, 6–22.

Sharkey, B.J. (2006). *Fitness and Health* 5th Edition. Champaign: Human Kinetics.

Szabo, A., (1995) The Impact of Exercise Deprivation On Well-being of Habitual Exercisers. *Australian Journal of Science and Medicine in Sport*. Vol. 27, 68–75.

The Sports Council and Health Education Authority (1992) *Allied Dunbar National Fitness Survey: Main Findings*. London: Sports Council and health Education Authority.

Chapter 9

Applied physiology for sports therapy

Introduction

Physiology is the study of how body systems work and integrate with each other across different contexts. Sport and exercise physiology is the study of how the body works applied to activity settings. More specifically it explains how the nervous, endocrine, musculoskeletal and cardiorespiratory systems work together to initiate and maintain movement, and to supply working tissues and remove waste products during activity.

The main aim of sports therapy is to optimise the performance of individuals and teams through the successful management of sport-related injuries. Therefore, a good grounding in physiology is vital as it underpins all work undertaken (for example how the body reacts and responds to being injured and the body systems involved in this). For a sports therapist a client's physiological state is a major determinant of sports performance, prehabilitation, mechanism of injury and adaptation to rehabilitation programmes. This chapter focuses on the key physiological principles that determine a sports therapist's work.

Learning outcomes

After you have read this chapter you should be able to:

- explain how aerobic capacity determines performance and injury
- explain how anaerobic power determines performance and injury
- describe adaptations to chronic training and conditioning
- explain physiological differences in clients
- explain the physiology of detraining.

Starting block

You have conducted a season-long injury audit with a local football team. When you start reviewing your data you notice that most injuries occurred at either the start of the second half or in the final ten minutes of the match.

- What reasons can you think of to explain this trend?

How aerobic capacity determines performance and injury

An individual's aerobic capacity determines their cardiorespiratory fitness. This is the body's ability to supply the working tissues with oxygen and how well these tissues can use this supply to maintain an active state. Many endurance-based sports, from triathlon to rugby league, require good levels of aerobic capacity for an athlete to perform well. However, many activities which are part of independent living also require basic levels of aerobic capacity, for example walking to the shops and climbing stairs.

If people have poor aerobic capacity it is associated with a poorer quality of life and an increased risk of chronic disease. For example, research has shown that low levels of aerobic power are linked to cardiovascular disease and depression in adults (Lee and Paffenbarger, 2000).

Understanding aerobic power will enable you to:

- preserve the health of clients (both with and without clear medical backgrounds)

- improve performance in clients across most sports

- ensure athletes return to sport fit and with a reduced risk of getting re-injured.

VO$_2$ max

The gold standard measurement of aerobic power is **VO$_2$ max**. Its definition suggests that each individual has a fictional aerobic power 'ceiling' and once this has been reached the body will start to **fatigue**. At what intensity an individual hits this fictional 'ceiling' or their VO$_2$ max will determine sports performance and risk of injury.

It is expressed absolutely in l/min or relatively using an individual's body mass as ml/kg/min. Elite endurance athletes may have VO$_2$ max values of 80+ ml/kg/min while adults with low levels of activity can have values below 20 ml/kg/min. In theory an athlete with a VO$_2$ max of 64 ml/kg/min will be able to perform better in endurance-based activity such as a 50 km cycle than an individual with a VO$_2$ max of 55 ml/kg/min. However, endurance performance is often also determined by who can perform longer at a higher percentage of their VO$_2$ max and psychology. For how you can test VO$_2$ max see *Chapter 6: Fitness testing for sports therapy*.

Key terms

VO$_2$ max – the maximum amount of oxygen the working tissues can extract and utilise during extreme exercise at sea level

Fatigue – general sensations of tiredness and an accompanying reduction in mental and physical performance

Remember

The sea level part of the VO$_2$ max definition allows research using VO$_2$ max data from all around the world and at different altitudes to be reliably compared.

If a specific sport requires the athlete to have an average VO$_2$ max score of 62 ml/kg/min to allow them to compete effectively, all athletes who fall below this requirement due to poor training or injury will not meet the demands of the sport, will fatigue early and face an increased risk of becoming injured.

Reaching VO$_2$ max

With steady state exercise (exercise where the intensity remains the same) oxygen consumption initially rises and then plateaus as the cardiorespiratory system gets used to meeting the stable demands of the exercise.

During incremental exercise (exercise where intensity increases with time) oxygen consumption by the working muscles keeps on increasing until it reaches the point where the muscles cannot consume any more oxygen to meet the increasing demands of the exercise. At this point the oxygen consumption will plateau based on the muscles working to their maximum capacity. The athlete has reached their VO_2 max and will need to stop exercising or reduce the intensity they are working at.

Other criteria which show that an athlete has reached their VO_2 max are:

- final exercise heart rate within 10 beats of **age predicted maximum**
- final exercise **lactate** concentration >8mmol/L
- final **respiratory exchange ratio (RER)** >1.15
- perceived exertion of greater than 19 using **BORG scale**
- subjective or volitional exhaustion.

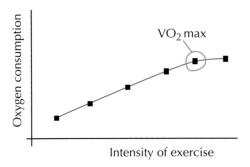

Figure 9.1: The relationship between oxygen consumption and incremental exercise

There are two major interlinking determinants of an athlete's VO_2 max and thus their cardiorespiratory endurance:

1. the chemical ability of the athlete's muscle tissues to use oxygen when breaking down carbohydrate, protein and fat for energy; associated with having to stop endurance-based exercise because muscles cannot function anymore

2. the combined ability of cardiovascular and respiratory systems to transport the oxygen to the working muscle tissues; associated with having to cease endurance exercise because of the body's inability to supply oxygen and remove carbon dioxide effectively, becoming too out of breath to continue.

The importance of carbohydrates

If an athlete competes and trains at a high percentage of their VO_2 max it is associated with extreme physiological changes that can affect performance and can increase the risk of injury (Shave and Franco, 2006). At rest an athlete obtains energy from mainly fat and a little carbohydrate. From approximately 70 per cent of an athlete's VO_2 max the body starts to rely more and more on carbohydrate as a source of fuel. Unfortunately the body can only store a limited amount of carbohydrate in the blood, liver and muscles. These stores are in the form of **glucose** in the blood or more importantly **glycogen** in the liver and muscles. Once glycogen stores start to reduce the body cannot use carbohydrate effectively for fuel, exercise feels harder and the body becomes fatigued. All of these together reduce endurance performance. For example, it generally takes 90 minutes working at 75 per cent VO_2 max for glycogen levels to reach a critical level.

Key terms

Glucose – a sugar that is the main form of carbohydrate used for fuel

Glycogen – stored carbohydrate in the liver and muscles

Age predicted maximum heart rate – theoretical maximum heart rate calculated by 220 minus age

Lactate – a salt formed from lactic acid

Respiratory exchange ratio (RER) – the ratio relating to volume of carbon dioxide expired to volume of oxygen consumed during activity

BORG scale – a scale of perceived exertion ranging from 6–20

Stop and think

During an endurance-based event what strategies could be used to prevent glycogen reaching a critical level?

The brain's only fuel source is carbohydrate; injuries to the athlete (and other competitors) may occur when carbohydrate sources run low. This is because brain chemistry is altered if an athlete works at a high percentage of their VO_2 max for a period of time. The hormone **serotonin** increases in the brain which makes an athlete feel tired, fatigued and lethargic. This can lead to poor concentration and decision making. For example, an athlete may make a mistimed tackle on an opponent causing injury.

Often endurance athletes may collapse or have to cease their performance based on 'hitting the wall'. This is associated with total physical and mental fatigue caused by the extreme demands of performing at a high percentage of VO_2 max. Once an athlete has 'hit the wall' they will not be able to continue and may require medical support.

How anaerobic power determines performance

Many sports require a good level of anaerobic power. For example, cycling up steep inclines, jumping, sprinting, kicking, lifting weights and punching all require **anaerobic power**. Anaerobic power can be defined as the ability to produce and maintain power output. The body cannot sustain anaerobic power output for very long before fatigue in the muscles builds up to a level where the athlete performs anaerobic movements at an increasingly poor level or stops altogether. For example, in karate, the power generated by punches and kicks will decrease at the end of a fight rather than at the start; in 100 metre sprinting the speed the athlete can generate at the start of the race will be greater than after fatigue has started to accumulate in the muscles at around 60 metres.

The fatigue associated with anaerobic power determines muscle performance and can increase the risk of injury (Wojtys, Wylie, and Huston, 1996). This could be why injuries in team sports that require sprinting, jumping and striking tend to be most commonly sustained towards the end of the game.

When an athlete is repeatedly required to perform powerful muscular movements they will undoubtedly fatigue. It is often those athletes who can maintain power output in the face of their muscles fatiguing that perform the best. Fatigue associated with anaerobic activities is thought to be caused by a number of interlinking factors (Wilmore, Costill, and Kenney 2008):

- alterations in energy delivery (**phosphocreatine (PCr)**, glucose)
- accumulation of waste products (heat, hydrogen ions, lactate)
- the nervous system's ability to contract working muscles.

When an athlete requires anaerobic power, the energy to be able to perform movement comes from PCr and the breaking down of glucose through anaerobic glycolysis. When these fuel sources start to become limited the muscles cannot produce enough **adenosine tri-phosphate (ATP)** to meet the demands of the activity and therefore cannot perform anymore.

Key terms

Serotonin – a hormone that causes changes in mood

Anaerobic power – the ability to produce and maintain power output

Phosphocreatine (PCr) – an energy-rich compound that plays a role in providing energy by maintaining ATP levels

Adenosine tri-phosphate (ATP) – a high energy phosphate compound that is the body's only direct source of energy

Fatigue, heat and lactate

Two waste products produced as a direct result of the muscles working are heat and lactate. High intensity activities or those requiring anaerobic power can produce a great deal of heat which raises the core temperature of both the muscles and the body. This rise in temperature causes fuel sources to be used more quickly and can result in key enzymes responsible for producing energy not working as effectively. Within the muscles a probable cause of fatigue is the build-up of lactic acid. It is not the lactic acid directly but what it breaks down into – lactate and specifically hydrogen ions – that cause fatigue. Movements requiring anaerobic power produce large amounts of lactate and hydrogen ions and subsequently lower the pH in the muscles. The drop in pH in the muscles stops the enzymes responsible for energy production working correctly. Without adequate recovery the lactate and hydrogen ions accumulate to a level where the muscle simply cannot perform sprinting, jumping or striking activities as well or at all. Lactate measurements are often taken as an indicator of muscle fatigue with high readings above 8 mmol/L associated with a major reduction in performance and exhaustion (Tesch, Sjodin, Thorstensson, and Karlsson, 2008).

Fatigue and neural stimulation of muscles

Fatigue that causes anaerobic power performance to reduce may also come from the nervous system's inability to maximally contract the muscles repeatedly. For a muscle to contract effectively a motor nerve must be able to stimulate the muscle fibres. This requires a **transmitter fluid** to carry the stimulus across a **neuromuscular junction**. Repeated anaerobic movements affect the transmitter fluid (too much or too little is produced) and the muscles simply cannot contract to their maximum potential any longer.

Fatigued muscles and possible mechanism of injury

As muscles fatigue due to repeatedly performing anaerobic power movements, the decrease in performance is associated with an increased risk of injury. Fatigue significantly reduces the amount of strength, speed and power the muscles can achieve. If the demands on the athlete remain the same throughout the duration of the sport then weaker muscles trying to meet these demands may become injured. For example, trying to out-jump an opponent in the fourth quarter in basketball with weak muscles may cause a muscle strain.

Key terms

Transmitter fluid – a fluid that allows a nerve impulse to be carried across a neuromuscular junction to enable a muscle contraction

Neuromuscular junction – the site where a motor nerve communicates with a muscle fibre

Activity

Measure yourself jumping as high as you can against a wall with a marker or time yourself running up a flight of stairs five times.

* What do you notice about the height you can reach or your time?
* What are the physiological mechanisms behind this?

One of the roles of muscles is to stabilise joints – weak muscles will not be able to stabilise joints effectively and can increase the risk of joint ligament injuries. An example to illustrate this would be trying to change direction quickly in extra time in football and the knee joint being stabilised by fatigued and weak muscle increasing the risk of knee ligament damage.

Adaptations to chronic training and conditioning

A key part of sports therapy work is returning athletes to full fitness or heightened levels of fitness post injury. *Chapter 7: Training and conditioning* covers the general theory behind why the body adapts following training, and the major training methods that can be used to improve specific components of fitness. This section focuses specifically on how the body adapts to various forms of training and conditioning.

Most training methods can be categorised into those that involve aerobic or anaerobic conditioning. Aerobic training methods are endurance based and improve central and peripheral blood flow and enable the muscle fibres to generate greater amounts of ATP. Anaerobic training methods are short duration/high intensity and improve high intensity endurance, and develop strength, speed and power. Table 9.1 shows the major physiological adaptations that you would expect to see in athletes engaging in aerobic training and conditioning.

Table 9.1: The major physiological adaptation of engaging in aerobic based training (the improvements in VO$_2$ max are caused by better cardiorespiratory and muscular functioning).

Physiological marker	Adaptations
Cardiorespiratory function	Cardiac **hypertrophy** (larger left ventricle); greater stroke volume, lower resting heart rate; faster recovery heart rate; increased blood volume; reduction in moderate/high blood pressure
Muscular function	More and more efficient **mitochondria**; more effective aerobic enzymes; better capillary supply for each fibre; greater storage of glycogen; more efficient type 1 fibres
Metabolic function	Oxygen consumption (VO$_2$ max) increases; athletes can operate with a higher lactate threshold
Body composition	Body fat reduces; bone density increases if the activity is weight bearing

(Adapted from Shave and Franco (2006))

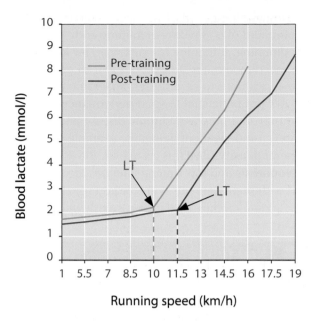

Figure 9.2: A graph to show the improvements in an athlete's lactate threshold (LT) following aerobic training and conditioning. If an athlete has a higher lactate threshold, how will this affect performance and risk of injury?

Table 9.2: The major physiological adaptation of engaging in anaerobic training

Physiological marker	Adaptations
Cardiorespiratory function	Cardiac hypertrophy (left ventricle becomes thicker); increased **stroke volume**
Muscular function	Better energy supply (PCr and glucose); more efficient anaerobic enzymes; muscle hypertrophy; more **motor units** are recruited; increase in power, speed and strength
Metabolic function	More lean tissue means that metabolic rate will be faster
Body composition	Greater amount of lean tissue; bone density increases if the activity is weight bearing

The short-term improvements in strength and power are caused by better neural factors, whereas long term improvements are caused by muscle hypertrophy (Wilmore et al., 2008).

Key terms

Hypertrophy – growth in size

Mitochondria – an organelle found in cells and the site of aerobic energy production

Stroke volume – the amount of blood ejected from the heart in one beat

Motor units – a motor nerve and all the muscle fibres it stimulates

Most physiological adaptations occur after a minimum of 6–8 weeks of training and conditioning. If training is maintained for longer, the magnitude of the adaptations will be greater. The adaptations to aerobic and anaerobic training are not just beneficial to sport performance but can also prevent injury and chronic disease and lead to longer independent living. For example, if **bone mineral density (BMD)** is increased, the risk of **osteoporosis** and low trauma fractures are reduced, and with improvements with cardiorespiratory functioning cardiovascular disease risk will be lower.

Key terms

Bone mineral density (BMD) – the density of bones determined by mineral content

Osteoporosis – accelerated deterioration of the weight bearing joints associated with ageing

Many athletes take part in both aerobic and anaerobic forms of training and conditioning activities and will adapt to both. For example, a rugby league player will train aerobically and anaerobically giving them a high VO_2 max while being able to generate high levels of power.

Each athlete will adapt at a different rate depending on race, gender, age, previous fitness levels and genetic background. There is a diminishing returns principle which reflects the fact that, the fitter you are, the harder it is to gain noticeable adaptations. For example, a previously inactive client starting to take part in aerobic based training will notice large improvements in their VO_2 max to begin with. As this client adapts and gains cardiorespiratory fitness the improvements in VO_2 max will become less noticeable. It is often the high level athletes who struggle to get any better than they currently are and can over train to the point of injury and illness.

Physiological differences in clients

As a sports therapist you may encounter a wide range of clients and athletes. Knowing about the physiological differences between these groups will enable more effective treatment, rehabilitation (early and late stage) and understanding about the mechanism of the injury.

This section will concentrate on the differences between:

- young (under 16 years) and older clients or athletes (50 years+)
- male and female athletes.

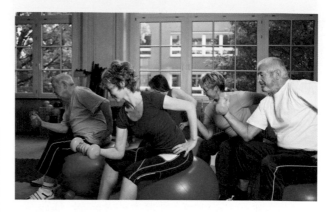

Figure 9.3: A group of middle aged adults taking part in a group-based resistance training session. In what ways will their age affect their adaptations to training and how would you reduce the risk of injury with these adults?

Younger clients

Younger clients' bones are not yet fully calcified and will not achieve this until they are in their early twenties. This means the whole of the skeletal system is underdeveloped. Growth plates on the epiphyses (ends) of long bones are not fused correctly and are particularly vulnerable as the skeleton is still growing. Muscles and bones develop at different rates in younger clients so care must be taken with muscular work and particularly maximal lifting as a number of muscles attach to key growth plates and over working these muscles can cause overuse injury and damage the growth plates and apophyseal injury. For example, Osgood-Schlatter disease is associated with overworking the quadriceps muscles and this results in repetitive traction on the tibial tuberosity. As the bones start to grow, the centre of gravity in young clients is affected so balance and co-ordination may become worse, especially in adolescence when they hit their peak growing velocity. Younger clients have underdeveloped anaerobic energy systems so any power or sprint-based training and conditioning will have very little impact and could in fact damage the immature skeleton if conducted too frequently.

For a position statement about training with under 16-year-old clients see the Rugby Football Union website. For a secure link to the site see Useful resources page 130.

Older clients

Many of the changes in older clients relate to body composition. Bone mineral density (BMD) reduces, particularly in post menopausal females, caused by reduced bone forming cell action and reduction in hormones responsible for nutrient absorption by the bones. Joint cartilage also deteriorates in the ageing process. This can mean older clients are at greater risk of fractures and osteoarthritis. Lean tissue tends to decrease by the process of **sarcopenia** leading to a reduction in strength, speed and power. This leads to a slower metabolism, increase in body fat and a slower recovery from exercise and injury. To offset these, older clients should try to maintain muscle function for as long as possible through conditioning work. Sprain and strain injuries may be more common based on reduced elasticity of muscle, tendons and ligaments. VO_2 max reduces by 10 per cent every decade post 20 years so older clients will be expected to have significantly reduced cardiorespiratory fitness (Wilmore et al., 2008). The risk of chronic diseases such as cardiovascular disease, diabetes type 2 and osteoporosis are subsequently higher in older clients.

Males and females

Physiological differences between males and females do not start until adolescence. When compared to females, males tend to be bigger, leaner and have more lean tissue. This is generally caused by the action of testosterone in males. This means males can generate more power, speed and strength. If females had the equivalent lean tissue of a male than many of these muscular differences would not be so evident. The VO_2 max of males also tends to be higher, thought to be caused by greater body fat and lower **haemoglobin** levels in females. As a result of the female sex hormones women tend to have more biomechanical faults than males. An example of this is due to wider hips and thus a greater **quadriceps angle (Q-angle)** places greater strain on joints when walking and running.

The menstrual cycle in females can make performance of exercise worse in those with pre-menstrual tension (PMT) and females may have low blood iron as a result of increased bleeding. For females athletes who compete in aesthetic sports (e.g. gymnastics and dance) or sports where there is an emphasis on leanness (endurance event, weight category sports), reducing body fat to a minimum through training and diet can lead to health issues. For example, low level of body fat can reduce the amount of oestrogen being produced and lead to **amenorrhea** and early onset osteoporosis (Yeager, Agostini, Nattiv, and Drinkwater, 1993).

> ### Key terms
>
> **Sarcopenia** – the process of lean tissue loss as we age
>
> **Haemoglobin** – an iron containing pigments that binds oxygen to red blood cells
>
> **Quadriceps angle (Q-angle)** – the angle between the line of the quadriceps muscle pull and the line of insertion of the patellar tendon
>
> **Amenorrhea** – absence of the menstrual cycle without being pregnant

> ### Stop and think
>
> If you suspect a female client has a critical level of body fat and you think that this is because of disordered eating and over training what would you do?

Physiology of detraining

Sustaining a sports injury usually means an athlete has to cease training for a period of time, or has to train at a lower intensity than normal. This can make an athlete anxious as their fitness levels will undoubtedly suffer as a result of the injury.

Detraining is defined as the partial or complete loss of training induced adaptation in response to stopping or lowering training intensity. In most cases sustaining a sports injury and subsequent losses in fitness are unavoidable. The losses in fitness and magnitude of the losses due to detraining depend on the severity of the injury and the length of time the athlete has to cease or lower training intensity. Unfortunately it is the more highly trained athlete who notices the greatest effects of detraining. The major effects of detraining on an athlete's fitness relate to:

- muscle strength, speed and power
- muscle endurance
- joint flexibility and proprioception
- cardiorespiratory endurance
- body composition.

Table 9.3: The major physiological effects of detraining on fitness

Fitness marker	Physiological changes
Muscle strength, speed, power	Muscle conditioning decreases within 2 weeks. In the short term this is associated with neural stimulation of muscles becoming worse. In the long term it is associated with muscle atrophy.
Muscle endurance	Within 2 weeks aerobic enzymes have reduced ability of up to 50 per cent. After 4 weeks glycogen content in the muscle is reduced by 40 per cent. Both of these explain the increased lactate production in muscle work and reduction in endurance.
Joint flexibility and proprioception	Both flexibility and proprioception are lost within a week both in and around the injured joint and others.
Cardiorespiratory endurance	VO_2 max decreases due to significant reductions (around 25 per cent) in cardiac output and reduced ability of aerobic enzymes with greater lactate production.
Body composition	The decrease in lean tissue lowers metabolic rate and can increase in overall body fat percentage. Often athletes will keep their eating behaviours when injured and may take in more calories due to low mood.

Remember

For most athletes, a few days away from training with an injury will not reduce fitness. In those who train intensively, the break may allow the body to repair and adapt thus improving performance.

Due to detraining a rehabilitation programme should aim to restore or enhance the athlete's fitness to where it was prior to injury. This can be done by following the IMPRESS acronym.

I – control and reduce inflammation

M – restore joint mobility and flexibility

P – restore proprioceptive ability

R – resistance training to restore strength

E – restore both cardiorespiratory and muscle endurance

SS – focus on sport specific functioning and attributes

Case study

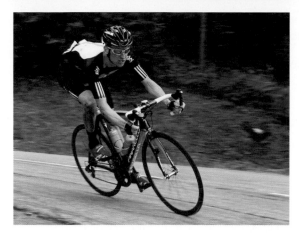

One of the most difficult endurance challenges in the world is the Tour de France. The Tour de France is an annual bicycle race held in France and nearby countries.

The race covers more than 3,600 km (2,200 miles) and lasts three weeks. The course involves a number of time trial and mountain-based stages. To win this race a cyclist must be able to meet the huge aerobic and anaerobic demands of the event.

1. What are the aerobic and anaerobic demands of the Tour de France?

2. How will a cyclist's body have changed due to training for this race?

3. What will be the mechanisms of fatigue during this race?

4. How will fatigue increase the cyclist's risk of injury?

5. What sort of injuries will the cyclist be at risk of and why?

 ## Check your understanding

1. Describe the term aerobic capacity.

2. Explain how an individual can tell if they have worked at their VO_2 max.

3. Explain which two mechanisms determine VO_2 max.

4. Describe the term anaerobic power.

5. Name sports that require high levels of anaerobic power.

6. Explain how fatigue can lead to the occurrence of injury.

7. What is the process of losing lean tissue as we age called?

8. What are the underlying reasons behind strength gains due to training?

9. What are the body composition differences between males and females?

10. Explain how having to stop training due to injury affects fitness levels.

To obtain answers to these questions visit the companion website at www.pearsonfe.co.uk/foundationsinsport

Useful resources

To obtain a secure links to the websites below, see the Websites section on page ii or visit the companion website at www.pearsonfe.co.uk/foundationsinsport.

Peak Performance Online
British Association of Sport and Exercise Sciences

Journal of Sports Science and Medicine

Sports Science – a peer-reviewed journal and site for sport research

Journal of Sports Sciences

Rugby Football Union training programmes

Further reading

Dick, F.W. (2007). *Sports Training Principles* 5th Edition. London: A&C Black.

Jeukendrup, A. and Gleeson, M. (2004). *Sports Nutrition*. Champaign: Human Kinetics.

Knight, K.L. and Draper, D.O. (2007). *Therapeutic Modalities: The Art and Science, with clinical activities manual*. Philadelphia: Lippincott, Williams & Wilkins.

Lee, L., and Paffenbarger, R.S. (2000) Associations of Light, Moderate, and Vigorous Intensity Physical Activity with Longevity – The Harvard Alumni Health Study. *American Journal of Epidemiology*. Vol. 151(3), 293–299

McArdle, W.D., Katch, F.I. and Katch, V.L. (2006). *Exercise Physiology: energy, nutrition and human performance*. Philadelphia: Lippincott, Williams & Wilkins.

Mohr, M., Krustrup, P. and Bangsbo, J. (2005). Fatigue in soccer: a brief review. *Journal of Sports Sciences*, Vol. 23, 593–599.

Nordstrom, A., Olsson, T. and Nordstrom, P. (2005). Bone gained from physical activity and lost through detraining: a longitudinal study in young males. *Osteoporosis International*, Vol. 16, 835–841.

Shave, R., and Franco, A., (2006) Chapter 4: The Physiology of Endurance Training. In Whyte, G. (2006). *The Physiology of Training: Advances in Sport and Exercise Science Series*. Philadelphia: Churchill Livingstone, Elsevier.

Tesch, P., Sjodin, B., Thorstensson, A., and Karlsson, J.,(2008) Muscle fatigue and its relation to lactate accumulation and LDH activity in man. *Acta Physiologica*.Vol. 103(4), 413–420

Whyte, G. (2006). *The Physiology of Training: Advances in Sport and Exercise Science Series*. Philadelphia: Churchill Livingstone, Elsevier.

Wilmore, J.H., Costill, D.L. and Kenney, W.L. (2008). *Physiology of Sport and Exercise* 4th Edition. Champaign: Human Kinetics.

Winter, E.M. et al (2007a). *The British Association of Sport and Exercise Sciences Guide: Sport and Exercise Physiology Testing Guidelines: Volume 1*. London: Routledge.

Winter, E.M. et al. (2007b). *The British Association of Sport and Exercise Sciences Guide: Sport and Exercise Physiology Testing Guidelines: Volume II: Exercise and Clinical Testing*. London: Routledge.

Wojtys, E.M., Wylie, B.B., and Huston, L.J., (1996) The effects of muscle fatigue on neuromuscular function and anterior tibial translation in health knees. *American Journal of Sports Medicine*. Vol. 24(5), 615–621

Yeager, K.K., Agostini, R., Nattiv, A., and Drinkwater, B., (1993) The female athlete triad: disordered eating, amenorrhea, osteoporosis. *Medicine and Sciences in Sport and Exercise*. Vol. 25, 7

Chapter 10

Biomechanics of sports injury

Introduction

Injury is a serious concern within public health and deserves the increased attention of sports therapists. It requires a multi and inter-disciplinary approach to prevention and treatment. Sports therapists adopt three perspectives to injury:

- **anatomical** – when they consider which tissues and structures have been injured
- **physiological** – when they understand the physiological and biological processes involved with tissue repair and recovery
- **psychological** – when they examine the cognitive, behavioural and social factors associated with injury risk and recovery.

Fundamental to each approach is the influence they have on sports performance. Biomechanics of sports injury focuses on the study of different factors (such as mechanical energy, footwear, equipment and surfaces) and their effects on sports performance. It is concerned with the way in which techniques are performed and has two functional roles: injury prevention and performance enhancement (with the latter incorporating biomechanical factors associated with rehabilitation). In essence, an understanding of the principles of biomechanics of sports injury is central to the work of any sports therapist. This is because it can be used to provide the basis for changes in technique, equipment or training routines that can help to prevent and rehabilitate injuries.

Learning outcomes

After you have read this chapter you should be able to:

- understand the term 'biomechanics'
- understand kinematic and kinetic influences on sports injury
- understand how Newton's laws of motion apply in a sports injury setting
- understand the uses of gait analysis in sports injury
- know the different methods of correcting abnormal biomechanics in sports therapy
- apply these principles to a case study and explain the causes of injury using biomechanical terminology.

Starting block

Have you ever watched two athletes, one who you think has a good technique and one who you think has a bad technique?

- What differences have you picked out in their techniques?
- How do you think these differences in technique could be linked to different sports injuries?

Biomechanics and kinetic and kinematic influences on sports injury

Biomechanics is the study of forces and their effects on living systems. In a sports injury context, you need to understand the different forces (both internal and external) that have played a role in the way that a sporting technique has been produced. Thus, you can also understand their role in a sports injury and the role that they will play in the rehabilitation of an injury.

Within biomechanics, there are two key terms: **kinematics** and **kinetics**. Kinematics in this context refers to the description of movements without reference to the forces involved, whereas kinetics refers to the assessment of movement with respect to the forces involved.

Kinematics

The kinematics of a movement involves an understanding of five primary variables (Whiting and Zernicke, 2008). These are as follows.

- **Timing of the movement** – the duration of force application that is associated with sports injury is often quite short (sometimes only a fraction of a second) but has high loading rates. This is an important factor to consider when looking at the causes of sports injury and injury rehabilitation.

- **Position or location** – the position of a body in relation to the forces being applied is an important consideration in explaining the causes of injury. For example, forces that are applied to the leg when it is flexed at the knee and externally rotated (as when controlling a football while the ball is in flight) will cause a

different type of injury from those forces applied to a leg when it is extended at the knee and flexed at the hip (as when following through on an instep kick).

- **Displacement** – when a body moves, its displacement is the movement in a straight line from point A to point B. This differs from distance when you look at how far something or somebody has had to move in any given direction to get from point A to point B. A body rotating about an axis experiences angular displacement which is measured in degrees of rotation or radians.

- **Velocity** – this is the rate of displacement. Linear velocity is calculated through linear velocity divided by the time taken whereas angular velocity is calculated by looking at the angular displacement divided by time.

- **Acceleration** – acceleration measures the rate of change of velocity. It has both linear and angular components.

Remember

Displacement, velocity and acceleration all play a role in understanding sports injury. Generally speaking, as each of these variables increase in magnitude, so does the severity of injury (for example, in a collision between two rugby players).

Kinetics

A kinematic analysis is an important factor in understanding any sports injury. However, as **force** is a causal factor in any injury, a kinetic analysis is also useful in understanding sports injury.

Key terms

Biomechanics – the study of forces and their effects on living systems

Kinematics – the description of movements without reference to the forces involved

Kinetics – the assessment of movement with respect to the forces involved

Force – mechanical action or effort applied to a body that produces movement

Force is the mechanical action or effort applied to a body that produces movement. It is measured in **Newtons**. A Newton is the force required to move a mass of 1 kg at a rate of 1m.s^{-2}. In sports therapy, you should have an understanding of the forces that are involved with a sports injury including:

- gravity
- **ground reaction forces**
- impact of objects
- compression forces exerted on long bones in lower extremities
- ligament forces acting on joints
- musculotendinous forces.

In instances where injuries are caused, there are seven factors that relate to force and will determine the severity of the injury (Whiting and Zernicke, 2008). These include:

- how much force is applied
- where the force is applied
- the direction of the force
- the time period for the application of the force
- how often the force is applied
- whether the force is constant or varied
- how quickly the force is applied.

Whenever an external force (also known as a **load**) is applied to a tissue, that tissue will experience a certain degree of **deformation**. As the load increases beyond the point of failure, the tissue will break or become damaged. Many traumatic injuries in sport tend to result from a **shear force** which, when the maximum capacity of **shear stress** is passed, will result in failure of the tissue. For example, if a player is tackled on the lateral aspect of the knee in football, the medial collateral ligament will experience a shear force and if that force is greater than the ligament can withstand, the ligament will tear (or fail under load). An interesting demonstration of the effects of shear force on bone tissue in a laboratory setting can be seen through Laycock, Smith and Liefeith (2006). (See *Further reading* on page 140.)

You should also bear the application of forces in mind when different gait and structural abnormalities are covered later in this chapter.

It is often the combination of these factors, and the gait or structural abnormalities, that will explain many injury causes when the injury is a non-traumatic injury.

Mass, inertia and torque

As well as the different factors that apply to forces, sports therapists must also include **mass**, **inertia** and **torque** when considering injuries.

A practical application of force, mass, inertia and torque can be seen in injuries sustained where rotation has occurred. In rapid twisting or turning movements such as tackles in football, or rapid changes of direction in rugby or basketball, the foot can sometimes remain in a fixed position. When this happens there is a certain amount of resistance to movement while at the same time the body is twisting, creating a large amount of torque through the joint (in this case the ankle and knee joints). When this rotational loading increases beyond the resistance to movement that the joint structures can maintain, one or more of the knee ligaments can be damaged. Furthermore, where the foot is plantar flexed and inverted in a fixed position, this can result in an ankle sprain affecting the anterior talo-fibular ligament or avulsion fractures of the lateral malleolus.

Key terms

Newton – force required to move a mass of 1 kg at a rate of 1m.s^{-2}

Ground reaction force – the equal and opposing force that is exerted by the ground on a body

Load – an external force

Deformation – a change in a tissue's shape when subjected to a load (deformation to failure means the amount of deformation of a tissue when it reaches failure)

Shear force – a force that often produces horizontal sliding of one layer of tissue over another

Shear stress – an internal resistance developed to a shear force

Mass – the quantity of matter in a body

Inertia – the resistance to changes in motion

Torque – the turning effect or twisting motion created by a force about an axis

How Newton's laws apply to a sports injury setting

Sir Isaac Newton identified laws of motion that are fundamental to the understanding of human movement. These laws can also be applied to a sports injury setting to help sports therapists explain the different mechanisms of injury. The application of these laws can be seen in Table 10.1.

Stop and think

Can you think of any other sports injury based examples of Newton's laws of motion?

Table 10.1: Newton's laws of motion and their application to sports injury

Law	Description	Application
Newton's First Law	A body will remain at rest (or in uniform motion) unless acted upon by an external force.	**A hard frontal tackle in rugby league.** Prior to the tackle, the player in possession of the ball will be sprinting at a given velocity. When the player is tackled, the outside force will rapidly decelerate or stop the player. For a short time, the player's head will obey Newton's First Law as it will keep travelling forwards, flexing the neck. The structures in the neck then prevent any further forward movement by resisting the forward motion thus causing rapid extension into hyperextension. This flexion – hyperextension pattern is typical of a cervical whiplash injury.
Newton's Second Law	A force acting on a body will produce an acceleration that is proportional to that force; as demonstrated through the equation force = mass × acceleration.	**A weightlifter attempting to dead lift 250 kg.** The body structures involved with the technique (e.g. quadriceps, knee joint) must be able to produce sufficient force to move the weight in an upward motion and must be able to resist the load that is placed upon them. If they are not able to produce the necessary force or withstand the load, they will become more susceptible to injury (e.g. muscle strain, ligament strain or cartilage tear)
Newton's Third Law	For every action there is an equal and opposite reaction.	**Ultra endurance athlete training for competition.** The concept of ground reaction forces is important in this scenario. Every time an ultra endurance athlete goes road running, they will be running for long periods of time. As the foot repeatedly strikes the floor, the ground exerts an equal and opposite force on the foot that acts through the lower extremities. Depending on the size, duration, frequency and rate of the force applied (as well as other factors such as footwear), this could result in overuse injuries such as stress fractures.

Gait analysis in sports therapy

This section covers the gait analysis of both walking and running, and the normal and abnormal biomechanics associated with gait. These are important considerations as they will often be the underlying cause of non-traumatic injury.

Biomechanics of walking

A walking normal gait contains a **stance phase** and a **swing phase** (these phases are shown in Figure 10.1). The stance phase begins and ends with a period where both feet are in contact with the ground where weight is being transferred from one foot to the other – known as **double support phase**. For the duration of each **gait cycle**, the foot is in stance position for 60 per cent of the time and in the swing phase for 40 per cent of the time.

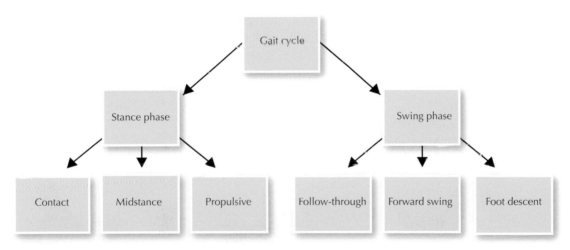

Figure 10.1: Elements of the gait cycle

Table 10.2 demonstrates the motion and position of the foot during a normal walking stance phase. An understanding of this phase is particularly important for injury prevention and rehabilitation as this is where the body will be experiencing the ground reaction forces that are a contributory factor in sports injury, particularly in those with an abnormal gait.

Table 10.2: The motion and position of the foot during the stance phase (N = neutral position)

	Contact	Midstance	Propulsive
Duration	27%	40%	33%
Motion	Pronation	Supination	
Position		Pronated	Supinated
	Heel strike	Foot flat	Heel off / Toe off

(adapted from Brukner and Khan, 2006)

Biomechanics of running

The biomechanics of running are broadly similar to those of walking in so far as running has the same stance and swing phases as walking. However, the key difference is that walking has a double support phase whereas running has a **flight phase**.

As running speed increases, so does the flight phase, meaning that somebody taking part in a 100 m sprint would have a longer flight phase than somebody running a marathon. Also, during different speeds of running, the foot mechanics change. During slower running, the foot maintains the same heel–toe pattern from contact to propulsion in the stance phase whereas during sprinting this changes so that the athlete maintains weight bearing through the forefoot from contact to propulsion. The differences in flight phase and foot contact patterns can be seen in Figure 10.2, with the shorter distance of the overall stride indicating a shorter stance phase and – therefore – a longer flight phase.

Abnormal biomechanics associated with gait

Abnormal biomechanics have been linked with a number of lower limb injuries in different populations. The main ones that affect the lower limb are foot over **pronation**, foot over **supination** and pelvic tilts. These abnormalities are described below, with lower limb injuries associated with the different abnormalities shown in Table 10.3 on page 138.

> ### Key terms
>
> **Flight phase** – the phase of the running gait where neither foot is in contact with the ground
>
> **Pronation** – eversion, dorsiflexion and abduction of the ankle joint
>
> **Supination** – inversion, plantar flexion and adduction of the foot

Over pronation

Over pronation causes injury because it leads to excessive internal rotation of the lower limbs during weight bearing activities, increasing the load on the different structures in the lower limbs. In addition, it can cause increased ground reaction forces on the medial aspect of the foot, increased load on the medial longitudinal arch and internal rotation of the tibia.

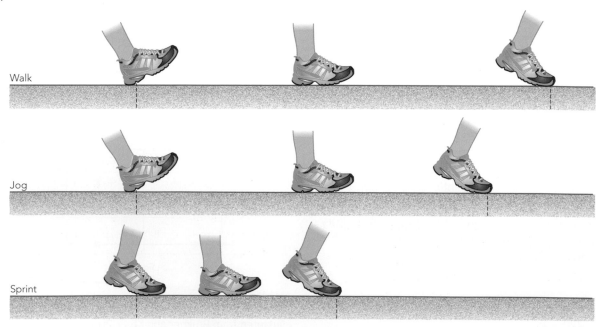

Figure 10.2: The differences between walking and sprinting
(Brukner, P. & Khan, K. (2006). *Clinical Sports Medicine*. McGraw-Hill Australia. p. 48)

Over supination

Over supination causes increased external rotational forces to act through the lower limbs, which places additional stress on the muscles and connective tissues in the lower limbs. Over supination is often caused by weakness in the muscles responsible for pronating the foot (the peroneal muscles), or as a result of tightness or spasms in muscles that supinate the foot (e.g. tibialis posterior, gastrocnemius and soleus). This condition usually causes overuse type injuries because a foot that over supinates often under pronates and, as pronation allows the foot to shock absorb, the stresses that are usually absorbed by the foot are absorbed by the lower limbs instead.

Activity

A simple test that can be used to assess your feet is the wet test. Visit the Runners World website for a demonstration and explanation of the wet test then complete it. How do your feet come out? See Useful resources on page 140 for a secure link.

Pelvic tilting

Anterior (pelvis tilting forwards) and lateral (pelvis tilting up or down on either side) pelvic tilts are both commonly associated with different sports injuries. Anterior pelvic tilts are caused by poor conditioning of the pelvic muscle (such as the gluteal muscles and abdominal muscles) whereas lateral pelvic tilts are usually caused by poor conditioning of the abductors and adductor muscles on the weight bearing limb.

Structural abnormalities

A knowledge of different structural abnormalities is important as they can result in a range of conditions and injuries (see Table 10.3). The key structural abnormalities in the feet and legs that are linked to different injuries are discussed below.

- **Forefoot varus** – a structural abnormality where the forefoot is inverted to the rear foot. The foot pronates excessively at the subtalar joint to allow the medial aspect of the foot to make ground contact.

- **Forefoot valgus** – a structural abnormality where the forefoot is everted to the rear foot. Supination occurs in the midtarsal joint and subtalar joint.

- **Rearfoot varus** – a structural abnormality where the calcaneus is inverted to the tibia which results in the subtalar joint excessively pronating to allow the medial aspect of the foot to make ground contact.

- **Rearfoot valgus** – a structural abnormality where the calcaneus is everted to the tibia due to the position of the subtalar joint. The midtarsal joint and subtalar joints supinate to attempt to compensate for this. This condition is the least common of the different structural abnormalities in the foot.

- **Bow legs** – this condition causes an increased varus heel strike which means that the body's main shock absorption system (the calcaneus) is not taking the ground reaction forces in an aligned position. As the impact is varus impact, this results in greater lateral stresses placed on the ankle and knee joints, as well as increasing the risk of pelvic tilts that can be the cause of back problems.

- **Knock knees** – these cause excessive pronation of the feet which results in a greater degree of medial stress being placed on the knee joint.

Remember

An understanding of the different structural abnormalities is essential for understanding most non-traumatic injuries.

Stop and think

Find images of each of the structural abnormalities and use the descriptions of each of the structural abnormalities relating to the foot, as well as the information earlier in the chapter relating to the role of forces, to discuss how the different conditions can result in different types of overuse injury.

Table 10.3: Lower limb injuries and associated gait and structural abnormalities

Injury	Potential biomechanical causes
Plantar fasciitis	Pronated foot
Achilles tendinopathy	Pronated foot
Medial shin pain	Pronated foot Varus alignment
Patellar tendinopathy	Pronated foot Anterior pelvic tilt Varus alignment
Patellofemoral pain	Pronated foot Anterior pelvic tilt Varus alignment
Stress fractures	Pronated foot Supinated foot
Hamstring strain	Anterior pelvic tilt
ITB syndrome	Anterior pelvic tilt Varus alignment

Different methods of correcting abnormal biomechanics in sports therapy

Once you have identified any key abnormalities in either gait or structure, one of your key roles is to look at how these can be corrected. Although this is within the professional limitations of the sports therapist for the most part, the client may need referring to a podiatrist for more specialist treatments (such as casted orthoses – see below). While it is outside the focus of this chapter to consider specific strength, proprioception, flexibility or core stability training (see *Chapter 7: Training and conditioning* for more details on these), they will be mentioned alongside the different biomechanical conditions to which they apply.

As the focus of the previous section was on gait and structural abnormalities, this section focuses specifically on methods of correcting these conditions – namely the use of orthoses, footwear, manual therapy techniques and training or conditioning methods.

Orthoses

Orthoses (also referred to as orthotics) are specialist insoles that are placed into footwear to help control excessive subtalar and midtarsal movements that may occur as a result of structural abnormalities. Orthoses are available as either preformed or casted orthoses. Preformed orthoses are available 'off the shelf', are more flexible in design and offer a limited degree of control over foot motion. Casted orthoses are produced from a plaster cast of the foot and are therefore tailored to the specific needs of the client. Casted orthoses are designed to significantly alter the foot mechanics and have a less flexible design than preformed orthoses.

When you are considering the use of orthoses, observe your client in their performance environment. This is because any structural or gait abnormality will usually react or manifest itself differently in a performance environment (as compared to a normal standing position or when walking). This is important as it will give you a better indication of how the body will react to the changes in posture and structure in a performance environment.

Remember

When deciding on the type of orthoses, consider factors such as the nature and severity of the abnormality, the client's body composition, their foot type and the type of sports or activity that they participate in.

Footwear

The wrong footwear is a major factor in injury, particularly in sports involving running, twisting or turning. While it is beyond the scope of this chapter to consider all aspects of all sports shoes commonly available, some generic themes can be discussed.

- It is important for all sports shoes to have a strong midsole that helps with shock absorption to reduce the risk of overuse injuries.

- Sports shoes should have a capacity for calcaneal cradling that supports and protects the heel to reduce the possibility of over pronation during sport and reduce the risk of associated injuries, as well as reducing the risk of bruising the heel.

- Assess the client's footwear for fit – ill-fitting footwear can result in blisters.

- A shoe that fits well but has insufficient padding in key areas could result in bursitis.

- The insole should have good shock absorption properties, should be able to absorb perspiration and should have an appropriate amount of friction to prevent the foot or sock sliding in the shoe.

Manual therapy techniques and training and conditioning methods

Abnormal gait or structural biomechanics are often rehabilitated using a range of different techniques. Earlier we looked at the different structural abnormalities and how they can lead to either lateral or medial stresses in the ankle knee and hip,

and how excessive pelvic tilts (lateral or anterior) can be linked to different injuries. You may find yourself using different massage techniques as well as different training and conditioning methods to help the rehabilitation process. Remember that, in the case of excessive pelvic tilts, they are often caused by either weakness, tightness or poor control in the muscles surrounding the pelvis. Here, your role would be to select and administer appropriate methods to meet the nature of the problem (for example, correct massage techniques, flexibility training, strength training and proprioception training (see Chapters 3, 4, 5 and 7 for more details about the different techniques and their associated benefits)).

Case study

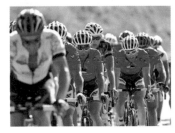

A cyclist was competing in a race. He broke his clavicle when he went over the top of his handlebars and struck his shoulder on the ground after being involved in a collision.

After the injury, the cyclist opted for surgical treatment of his fracture and the clavicle was repaired with a plate and a number of screws.

The time that clavicle fractures take to heal varies with age, health, complexity and the location of the break as well as the bone displacement. Eight weeks is a normal approximation of recovery time. With surgical stabilisation

of the bone, activities such as cycling can resume more quickly. The potential risks of surgery include risks of infection, nerve injury, or the plate used to fix the clavicle can be uncomfortable and may need to be removed.

1. Research this type of injury so that you have a detailed understanding of the injury and the recovery. Lance Armstrong suffered this type of injury when competing in the Vuelta of Castilla and Leon Stage Race and articles and videos are available for research about this.

2. How can you explain this type of injury using biomechanical reasoning?

3. Why is an understanding of the biomechanics behind this type of injury important for a sports therapist when considering the rehabilitation plan?

Check your understanding

1. What is biomechanics and how does it apply in a sports injury context?

2. What do the terms kinetics and kinematics mean?

3. What are the force-related factors that can affect injury?

4. What is the relationship between external force and traumatic injury?

5. What are Newton's laws of motion?

6. What is the normal walking gait cycle?

7. What is the key difference between walking gait and running gait?

8. What are the abnormal biomechanics that are associated with gait?

9. What are the common foot structural abnormalities?

10. What are orthoses and how can they help foot biomechanics?

To obtain answers to these questions visit the companion website at www.pearsonfe.co.uk/foundationsinsport

Useful resources

To obtain a secure link to the websites below, see the Websites section on page ii or visit the companion website at www.pearsonfe.co.uk/foundationsinsport.

Virtual Sports Injury Clinic

Sports Injury Bulletin

SportEx

Take the Wet Test: Learn Your Foot Type – article from *Runner's World*

Further reading

Bartlett, R. (1999). *Sports Biomechanics: Reducing Injury and Improving Performance.* London: E&FN Spon.

Blazevich, A. (2007). *Sports Biomechanics: The Basics: Optimising Human Performance.* London: A&C Black.

Brukner, P. and Khan, K. (2006). *Clinical Sports Medicine* 3rd Edition. North Ryde: McGraw-Hill.

Laycock, R., Smith, A. and Liefeith, A. (2006). Breaking Bones: Animating the Biomechanics of Sport Injury. *Journal of Hospitality, Leisure, Sport and Tourism Education*, Vol. 5, 77–83.

Whiting, W.C. and Sernicke, R.F. (2008). *Biomechanics of Musculoskeletal Injury* 2nd Edition. Champaign: Human Kinetics.

Chapter 11

Psychology of sports injury

Introduction

Sports injuries happen for different physical, psychological and sport-specific reasons. Although the hands-on work of sports therapists focuses predominantly on the physical and sport-specific injury risk factors, sports therapists also have a role to play in the psychological elements of rehabilitation. Due to the increased incidence of sports injury, and the greater recognition of the role psychology plays in the sports injury experience of athletes, sport psychology has become an important avenue for sports therapists to explore.

How quickly and how well an athlete reacts to their sports injury has huge implications for the speed of their recovery. An athlete that is motivated and makes positive and informed decisions about their recovery process and rehabilitation period is more likely to have a successful rehabilitation and return to sport than one who stalls on the negative aspects of injury. Reframing the injury period as a challenge that athletes must overcome to be successful in sport, rather than approaching the injury as something that can threaten their career, is something that you must be able to do to help your client through the recovery process.

Throughout this chapter you will learn about the sports injury experience of athletes, from the different factors that can predispose the athlete to injury to how you can facilitate a smooth return to performance. An underlying theme is recognising your professional limitations of practice as a sports therapist and ensuring that you only work within your areas of competence when taking on the challenge of the psychological element of the rehabilitation of injuries.

Learning outcomes

After you have read this chapter you should be able to:

- understand psychological factors associated with the occurrence of sports injury
- understand athlete responses to sports injury
- know the different signs of poor adjustment to injury
- understand psychological factors associated with sports injury rehabilitation adherence
- understand different interventions used in sports injury rehabilitation
- understand psychological factors associated with the return to sport.

Starting block

Do you know somebody who has had an injury that has kept them out of their sport or exercise for a period of time? What changes happened during their period of injury? How much of it do you think could be attributed to their responses to the injury?

Psychological factors associated with the occurrence of sports injury

Sports injuries are commonly linked to some form of stressor. Williams and Andersen (1998) produced a stress injury model (see Figure 11.1 on page 143) that demonstrates the link between potentially stressful events and sports injuries. The main theme is that athletes who have a combination of:

- a history of **stressors**
- personality characteristics that can make stressful situations worse
- few coping resources to deal with stress

are more likely to get injured.

This is because they will see a potentially stressful event (e.g. an important match) as more threatening and will experience greater physiological changes (e.g. hyper-elevated muscle tension) and psychological changes (e.g. concentration disruption, narrowing of the visual field). Increased muscle tension caused by stress can result in increased muscle fatigue and reduced flexibility, which can reduce the quality of technique and result in an increased risk of injuries such as strains and sprains. Concentration disruption and narrowing the visual field could lead to missing important information about game play. For example, not noticing a player coming in to tackle, which means the athlete may not be able to prepare themselves for impact or adjust their body position to avoid it. It is the severity of these physiological and psychological changes that predisposes athletes to injury. The final part of this model suggests that

Key term

Stressor – something that causes you stress, for example an injury

adequately planned interventions reduce the risk and severity of injury in athletes.

History of stressors

Stressors include stressful life events, daily hassles, sport-specific issues and previous injuries. The greater the life stress that an athlete experiences (both sporting and non-sporting) the greater the severity and incidence of injury (Johnson and Ivarsson, 2011; Patterson, Smith and Everett, 1998; Steffen, Pensgaard and Bahr, 2009) with injuries likely to occur 2–5 times more frequently in athletes with high life stress than in those with low life stress (Williams and Roepke, 1993).

Remember

Previous injury is a key stressor that can influence future injury (Walker et al., 2007). Athletes who are worried about the recurrence of a previous injury or their state of recovery are more susceptible to re-injury because they are more easily distracted and less focused during competition.

Personality factors

Certain personality characteristics can reduce the risk of injuries because they help the client to perceive situations as less stressful or threatening. Conversely, relationships have been found between injury and competitive trait anxiety, low self-esteem and negative mood states. However, most research that has examined personality variables as an injury risk factor has produced mixed results (e.g. Kolt and Kirby, 1996). This is partly due to the lack of sports-specific personality measures.

Coping resources/behaviours

Compared to personality factors, high coping resources (ways of dealing with stressors) and coping behaviours (using coping resources to deal with stressors) have received less research attention in sports injury research, but have produced more consistent results (Williams and Scherzer, 2010). High coping resources and coping behaviours are linked to a decreased occurrence of injury due to a decreased stress response to potentially stressful situations.

There are three main types of coping resource used by athletes:

1. **avoidance coping** – where the client doesn't acknowledge there is a problem, e.g. denial, wishful thinking

2. **emotion-focused coping**, e.g. imagery, social support

3. **problem-focused coping**, e.g. goal setting, gathering information.

Of the different coping resources available to athletes, social support has been highlighted as a key factor in the rehabilitation of sports injury (Petrie, 1993; Udry, 1996; Walker, Thatcher and Lavallee, 2007). Social support comes from family, friends, partners, teammates, coaches, support staff and even religious groups. There are three different aspects to social support:

- **emotional support** – listening, emotionally comforting or challenging somebody

- **informational support** – expressing appreciation for hard work, providing Information about performance and motivating people to achieve even more, e.g. 'Well done, you're on the right track so let's keep it going now and keep working towards recovery.'

- **tangible support** – providing material and personal support.

Remember

Because social support helps to reduce the incidence of injury and because of its benefits during injury rehabilitation, you should recommend that your client seeks social support from both sporting and non-sporting settings.

Cognitive appraisal

The stress injury model shown in Figure 11.1 suggests the way that an athlete perceives a potentially stressful event is affected by their personality factors, the available coping resources and their coping behaviours. If an athlete sees a potentially stressful situation as challenging (facilitative), rather than threatening (debilitative), their risk of injury is reduced. This is because the behaviours that the athlete will display during training and competition will be more positive. As a sports therapist, you need to understand that the way an athlete perceives a situation can change over time and should try to guide your client towards viewing the positive, challenging elements of any potentially stressful situation.

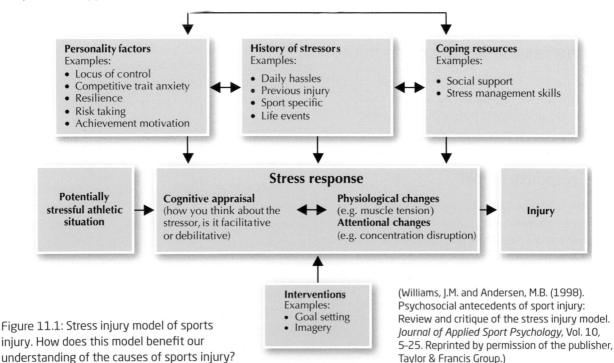

Figure 11.1: Stress injury model of sports injury. How does this model benefit our understanding of the causes of sports injury?

(Williams, J.M. and Andersen, M.B. (1998). Psychosocial antecedents of sport injury: Review and critique of the stress injury model. *Journal of Applied Sport Psychology*, Vol. 10, 5–25. Reprinted by permission of the publisher, Taylor & Francis Group.)

Cognitive appraisal – the way that we think about potentially stressful situations. This is linked to personality characteristics that influence the rehabilitation process and situational factors (sport, social and environmental factors that can influence injury rehabilitation)

Other factors related to the occurrence of sports injury

The attitudes of those involved with athletes, such as coaches and team managers, can increase the risk of injury, for example, 'Go tough, or go home!', 'No pain, no gain' and 'If you're injured, you're useless to me!'.

This is because they encourage a culture of playing through pain, making the athlete feel like they are only worth something if they can play in a winning team and persuading athletes to take unnecessary risks in competition. Sports coaches, sports therapists and team managers should help athletes to realise that they still have a role to play in the team even if they are injured and reinforce this with appropriate behaviours. They should make a point of helping athletes to distinguish between what is normal training discomfort as opposed to over-training.

Athlete responses to sports injury

Despite the best efforts of everybody involved with sport, injuries are inevitable. As a sports therapist, you need to understand how athletes react to injuries so that you can help plan the best course of rehabilitation.

Grief response model

An early way of understanding psychological responses to sports injury came through the grief response model (see Table 11.1). This is a stage model that was originally designed by Kübler-Ross (1969) to understand the grieving process but has since been applied to sport injury. The model outlines clear stages as shown below.

Table 11.1: Stages of grief response with example thoughts and behaviours

Stage of reaction	Thoughts	Behaviours
Denial – where athletes find it hard to accept that they are injured	I can play my way through this injury. It won't stop me.	Continue to play or train with injury
Anger – which can be directed at the injury, support staff or oneself	Why did the coach make me play that new position? Just my luck to get injured before the finals!	Storm away from training or a team meeting
Bargaining – where the athlete almost makes a deal with themselves about how to rehabilitate	If I do all the exercises at home maybe I can play next week earlier than expected. They don't really know how athletes feel.	Failure to follow medical advice regarding rest and rehabilitation
Depression – where athletes demonstrate sadness and apathy towards the injury and rehabilitation process, often believing that they will not get better	I'm not getting anywhere with this exercise programme. Why should I even bother going to rehab?	Lack of motivation, lethargy, withdrawal
Acceptance – where the athlete finally accepts that they are injured and the only way forward is to work through the rehabilitation process.	I can now see that the sports therapist was right. I should continue to follow their advice.	Positive self-talk, commitment/ adherence to rehabilitation

Although regularly cited in sports injury literature, the grief response approach has been criticised (see Brewer, 1994; Walker et al., 2007 for critical reviews) because of its sequential nature, suggesting that all injured athletes go through these stages in this order. However, some athletes may not even demonstrate some of these emotions during the injury period. You should look on this model as something that can help you to understand emotional responses to injury that athletes *may* go through.

Cognitive appraisal model of sports injury

The cognitive appraisal model of sports injury (Brewer, 1994) gives us an accepted way of understanding responses to sports injury. This approach suggests that the athlete views their injury as a stressor which they then evaluate based on different situational factors including:

- sport-related factors, e.g. the part of the season that the injury occurred in
- social factors, e.g. the influence of their coach
- environmental factors, e.g. access to rehabilitation opportunities
- different personal factors, e.g. a history of successful rehabilitation from injury, motivation and pain tolerance.

The way that the athlete evaluates their injury then determines their emotional response (e.g. anger, relief) which then determines their behavioural response (e.g. how well they adhere to rehabilitation programmes).

Three categories of response

Udry, Gould, Bridges and Beck (1997) suggested three categories of response that all athletes go through during the injury period (some moving through them more quickly than others).

1. **Injury relevant information processing stage** – where the injured athlete wants information about the injury such as recovery time and the nature of the pain. This stage has the greatest negative emotions. The main concern for the athlete is the inconvenience that the injury causes to their everyday life.

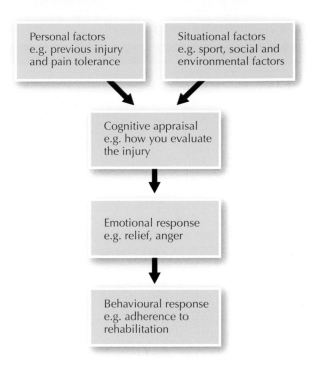

Figure 11.2: Cognitive appraisal model of psychological adjustment to sports injury. How do you think each of the sections can influence injury rehabilitation?

(Brewer, B.W. (1994). Review and critique of models of psychological adjustment to athletic injury. Journal of applied sport psychology, Vol. 6, 87–100. Reprinted by permission of the publisher (Taylor & Francis Group, http://www.informaworld.com).)

2. **Emotional upheaval and reactive behaviour stage** – where the athlete becomes emotionally agitated and irritable, and emotionally and physically tired. The athlete might isolate themselves from others while being in denial and despair about the injury.

3. **Positive outlook and coping stage** – where the athlete begins to accept that they are injured and starts to deal with the injury. They demonstrate a more positive outlook and attitude towards the recovery process because they begin to get a sense of progress.

There are also other, more general responses to injury that you need to know when working as a sports therapist. These are outlined in Table 11.2.

Table 11.2: Different reactions to injury

Reaction	Examples
Concerns over reduction in performance levels	Athletes often have trouble reducing expectations about their own performance and find it difficult to accept that they cannot perform at their pre-injury levels immediately post injury. Sports therapist and support team must make sure that athletes are aware that drops in performance are normal due to changes during the injury period (e.g. weight gain, reduction in important components of fitness, missed training time and missed competition time). Work towards helping the athlete understand when/how they should be able to expect to return to pre-injury levels of performance.
Fear	When injured, athletes spend a lot of time not being able to train or compete, which means that they spend a lot of time thinking about the injury. When they do this, they can experience fear, e.g. of re-injury or being replaced in their squad, team or rankings.
Decreased confidence	When an athlete cannot play or train, they start to lose confidence in their abilities. This, combined with the physical changes that occur during the injury period, can lead to the athlete losing motivation to rehabilitate, concentration being disrupted or re-injury.
Identity loss	When injured, athletes can lose their sense of identity because they cannot compete. This can be a particularly significant reaction for those who suffer career ending injuries.

The different signs of poor adjustment to injury

The theoretical approaches outlined above suggest that the athlete will go through a number of emotional changes throughout the injury period. Athletes will respond differently to injuries, some of them worse than you expected. You need to be aware of the warning signs that the athlete is adjusting to their injury experience poorly so that you can provide the correct support.

The following signs and symptoms are suggested by Petitpas and Danish (1995) as markers of the athlete responding badly to the sports injury:

- anger and confusion
- obsession with returning to play
- denial through repeatedly suggesting that the injury isn't a big problem
- returning to injury too soon and repeatedly re-injuring as a result
- paying too much attention to minor problems
- feeling guilty about letting the team down
- mood disturbance and rapid mood swings
- isolating or withdrawing oneself from significant others
- believing that they will never recover
- overemphasis placed on minor achievements.

Recognise your limitations of practice and the scope of your competence. You may need to refer your client to a sports psychologist or another mental health professional so that they can get the support that they need.

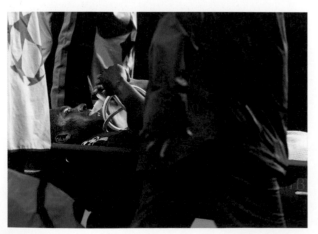

Figure 11.3: Antonio Valencia suffered a broken and dislocated ankle and severe ligament damage in the 2010/11 season. The football player was out of action for the majority of the season. How might a player react psychologically following such a serious injury? How do you think you could help?

Whether your client is struggling to adjust to injury or not, the road to recovery is often long and difficult for athletes so you should be aware of the different factors that influence rehabilitation adherence in injured athletes.

Psychological factors associated with sports injury rehabilitation adherence

You must find ways to ensure that your client sticks to a rehabilitation programme that may include several sessions, changes to diet and nutritional patterns, home exercises, intensive training programmes in the later stages of functional rehabilitation and psychological skills training activities. When designing these programmes, involve your client so that they feel more in control. This will also lead to improved communication, an efficient working relationship and increased rehabilitation adherence.

One way to maximise the rehabilitation adherence of your client is to identify the factors that determine it. These factors have been classified by Crossman (2001) under three headings, as follows.

- **Predisposing factors** relate to the client's views about the recovery process. Ask the client how they think they will achieve their goal of regaining competitive fitness. In this way you can guide them towards thinking about factors in the rehabilitation programme that will influence their recovery and help them to recognise the importance of the programme.

- **Reinforcing factors** are based on how the client interacts with significant others around them. Ask questions such as 'Are you staying in contact with your coaching staff?' This encourages your client to understand the importance of the support team and of using all the available support mechanisms to help them through the rehabilitation process. It will also help your client to understand the impact that their recovery can have on other people and stress the importance of rehabilitation adherence from an alternative perspective.

- **Enabling factors** help the client to attend the rehabilitation programme (or there may be factors that prevent them from attending). Ask questions such as 'What other commitments do you have outside your rehabilitation programme?' and 'Is there anything that can be done to make it easier for you to attend?' This is an important stage as it helps you to identify (with your client) factors that enable them to attend rehabilitation.

Within the predisposing, reinforcing and enabling factors, you could consider personal and situational factors that influence rehabilitation adherence (see Table 11.3). The ideal rehabilitation situation for any injured athlete is that they have optimal personal characteristics and a comfortable, convenient environment for their rehabilitation programme.

Table 11.3: Personal and situational factors associated with sports injury rehabilitation

Personal factors	Situational factors
Pain tolerance	Belief in the rehabilitation process and procedures
Mental toughness	
Self-motivation	Comfortable environment
Independence	Convenient appointments
A master goal orientation	Appropriate exertion levels
	Social support

Brewer (1998) provided a list of behaviours that are typical of injured athletes who are adhering to their rehabilitation programmes appropriately including:

- following instructions to restrict activity

- completing home exercises without fail

- completing home self-therapy (such as icing the injury)

- taking prescribed medication as expected

- enthusiastic and consistent participation in the rehabilitation programme.

Different interventions used in sports injury rehabilitation

Stop and think

What do you think are your limitations of practice where psychological skills training and the counselling of injured athletes are concerned?

When working as a sports therapist, you may not have a background or in-depth training in the psychology of sports injuries. The following recommendations will help when you are thinking about the psychological aspect of work with clients.

- Recognise the limitations of your practice.

- Have in place a referral network of appropriate professionals, such as sports and exercise psychologists.

- Attend formal training courses and workshops on sports psychology, psychological skills training, counselling approaches adopted within sports psychology and their role in sports injury prevention and rehabilitation.

- Shadow other professionals working with injured athletes so that you can learn to recognise the signs of poor adjustment to injury, how to deal with athletes with long-term or career-ending injuries and to learn about different coping resources/behaviours adopted by injured athletes.

Be prepared for your client to demonstrate frustration, anger, disbelief and denial throughout the injury period. These emotions make it difficult for injured athletes to develop a relationship with support staff, but you can aid the process by following these suggestions.

- Remain positive about the injury recovery process, but always be honest with your client and do not be overly optimistic. Being too optimistic can lead to unrealistic expectations and could result in a poor working relationship or increased risk of re-injury.

- Develop a team approach to recovery (i.e. you and the athlete are in it together) so that the athlete does not feel isolated.

- Show empathy for the injury but do not be overly sympathetic as this can seem patronising.

- Be a social support mechanism for the athlete on an emotional and informational level. Especially in the case of long-term injuries, you will be the person who the athlete sees the most in the club so you will be best suited to provide this level of support. However, make sure that you also foster social support with other aspects of the team set-up (e.g. ensure there is a presence from other coaching staff and players when appropriate).

Heil (1993) suggested four distinct groups of techniques that can be used to help rehabilitate clients:

- education

- goal setting

- social support

- psychological skills training.

Education

Educate the client on what to expect during the injury and rehabilitation process, especially if this is their first injury. This increases their sense of control and active participation. When they understand the recovery process, they can commit to rehabilitation and are more likely to put effort into it. Educate athletes about the emotional difficulties that they are likely to experience and teach them about the importance of rehabilitation adherence, particularly looking at the effects of lack of effort or over-motivation.

You should also educate clients about the nature of the injury. An understanding of the anatomy, physiology and healing process related to the injury, combined with information about the rehabilitation process, will help the client to make informed decisions about their goals, their risk taking and their personal safety upon return to training and competition.

Finally, clients should be taught to differentiate between different types of pain. It is important that the client can recognise the difference between dangerous pain (injury) and benign pain ('normal' pain experienced through the rehabilitation process).

Stop and think

Why is it important to educate the athlete about the sports injury and the rehabilitation process?

Goal setting

This is an essential element of rehabilitation and can be informed by the education process during the early stages of injury. It increases motivation, the amount of effort put into rehabilitation sessions and home exercises, directs attention towards specific aspects of recovery and has been linked to faster recovery.

You should work with your clients to develop a combination of short-term and long-term goals as well as developing a combination of **performance**, **process** and **outcome goals**.

Key terms

Performance goal – a goal that focuses on achieving performance objectives independent of other athletes

Process goal – a goal that focuses on the actions that an individual must undertake to perform well

Outcome goal – a goal that focuses on the outcome of an event

All goals should follow the SMARTS acronym (Smith, 1994):

Specific – goals say exactly what needs to be done

Measurable – goals are quantifiable and evaluated on a regular basis

Action orientated – the client will have to do something to achieve the goal

Realistic – the goals are within the constraints of the injury and stage of rehabilitation

Time orientated – goals have a time frame for completion that is realistic for the client

Self-determined – goals are either set by, or have an input from, the client so that the client feels more 'in control' and less like they are just being told what to do.

Activity

Choose a long-term injury for a sport of your choice (e.g. an anterior cruciate ligament rupture in a rugby union player).
- Research the rehabilitation plan and recovery process for this type of injury.
- Produce a goal setting plan to help guide the client through the recovery process.

Social support

As already stated, you will be an important provider of social support, but it will also come from friends, family, teammates and coaches. Social support can reduce injury-related stress levels and increase motivation to rehabilitate and rehabilitation adherence (Bianco and Eklund, 2001). Teammates and coaches need to understand that the injured athlete can feel isolated, so it is essential that they maintain contact. Ongoing contact also helps to maintain the athlete's confidence that they will be able to return to the team. Support from other athletes who have experienced similar injuries and recovered can be particularly beneficial. It can help them to see that recovery is possible and reduce levels of despair and anxiety, as well as having somebody who can educate them about the injury and recovery experiences from a first-hand perspective.

Psychological skills training

This is used by athletes during rehabilitation to minimise the psychological effects of injury and to increase confidence that they will be able to return to competition. The different psychological skills used reduce some of the physical symptoms of injury and offer the injured athlete the opportunity to take part in sport-specific training (albeit psychological sport-specific training) during a time that is normally considered by the athlete as enforced 'time away' from all sporting activity. The benefits of psychological skills training are shown in Figure 11.4.

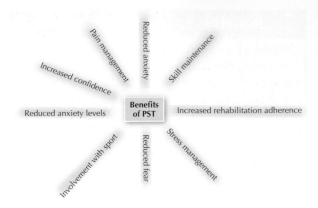

Figure 11.4:The benefits of psychological skills training during injury rehabilitation

Imagery

Imagery is an important part of rehabilitation (Cupal and Brewer, 2001; Dreidiger, Hall and Callow, 2006). It aids the healing process, offers an opportunity for practice during the injury period and can increase rehabilitation adherence (Ievleva and Orlick, 1991). It has also been shown to be a coping strategy that is used by athletes who successfully rehabilitate from injury more than those who are unsuccessful (Udry et al., 1997).

When educating your athlete about imagery, consider the following points.

- Imagery is a skill and like any skill it takes time to develop it.
- The client should use an imagery perspective (**internal** or **external**) that is most natural for them.
- Images should use all of the senses and different emotions.
- Images used should have vivid experiences.
- The athlete should be taught to develop imagery control to prevent 'spontaneous' images of the injury occurring.
- Images should consider physiological and psychological factors in rehabilitation.

Key term

External imagery – imagining yourself doing something as though you are watching it on a film so that you can develop an awareness of how the activity looks

Internal imagery – imagining yourself doing something and concentrating on how the activity feels

Table 11.4: Types of imagery used in rehabilitation. Why do you think it is important to have a good knowledge of each of the different types and their benefits?

Table 11.4 shows different types of imagery used during rehabilitation, the associated processes and outcomes of the different types of imagery.

Type	Use	Process	Associated outcomes
Healing imagery	Healing process	Images of healing process (e.g. increased flow of blood to injured area)	Increased confidence in rehabilitation Stress reduction Pain management
Pain imagery	Pain management	Images of factors causing pain then pain reducing Images of athlete handling the pain	Increased confidence in rehabilitation Stress reduction Pain management
Relaxation imagery	Relaxation/pain management	Calming images (e.g. relaxing on a sunny beach)	Distraction from pain Pain management Stress reduction
Performance imagery	Maintains skill levels Makes athlete feel 'involved' with their sport still Non-physical training that can benefit athlete on return to performance	Images of athlete performing skills correctly, can be more effective if done in a familiar environment that is related to sport (e.g. on the pitch)	Skill maintenance/enhancement Attention distraction Increased confidence in rehabilitation outcome Pain management Stress reduction

Activity: Relaxation imagery

Read through this imagery script, imagining yourself in the scene.

Imagine that you are on a beach. It is beautiful. You can feel the warm sun on you. You can see the golden sands where they meet the clear blue waters. Up above you can see the blue sky. It is clear with a couple of white fluffy clouds. You are now walking towards the water and you can feel the sand between your toes as you walk. You can hear the waves roll in and break at the shore line as you get closer to the water's edge. The water starts to splash against you and you can feel the cooling effect of the water on your skin. You are now stepping into the water and you feel the cool sensation on your feet and then on your legs as you walk in deeper. You dive into the water and enjoy the cooling sensation. Everything is peaceful, there are no sounds except for the water and as you swim you can feel the warm sun on your back. You are completely at peace, calm, warm and relaxed.

- How did you feel at the end of the script?
- How well did you image the scene?
- How do you think this type of script could benefit injured athletes?

Progressive muscular relaxation (PMR)

Muscle tension can lead to an increased risk of injury or re-injury due to vastly decreased flexibility and poor co-ordination. Progressive muscular relaxation (PMR) is an easy-to-use technique that helps to reduce muscle tension. It raises awareness of levels of muscle tension and, through the relaxation phase, helps the client to distinguish between what is a state of tension and relaxation. The technique involves tensing and relaxing groups of muscles in turn over the whole body. Each muscle group is tensed for five seconds, the tension is then released for five seconds, a deep breath is taken and the process is repeated. It is called progressive muscular relaxation because an athlete progresses from one muscle group to the next until all muscles have been tensed and relaxed.

Self-talk

When injured, an athlete can start to have negative thoughts. They may start to place too much emphasis on pain which can increase their perceptions of pain levels; this can force them to reduce activity levels and can reduce motivation to adhere to rehabilitation. All of this increases the rehabilitation time. As a sports therapist, you could help them to learn to talk to themselves more positively during the rehabilitation period. **Positive self-talk** can help the client manage their emotional response to the injury, increase their motivation and adherence to the rehabilitation programme and direct their attention towards specific elements of the programme. Figure 11.5 demonstrates the impact that changing **negative self-talk** to positive self-talk can have on the emotional and behavioural responses to injury.

Key term

Positive self-talk – positive statements used to arouse and direct attention or to motivate people towards achieving goals

Negative self-talk – self-critical statements that can distract attention, reduce confidence and self-efficacy levels and make it harder to achieve goals

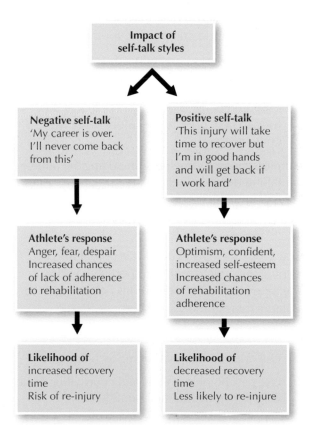

Figure 11.5: Examples of negative and positive self-talk statements resulting from serious injury. What other types of statements do you think athletes would make and how could you turn those into positive statements?

Psychological factors associated with the return to sport

On returning to sport, athletes often report a number of different stressors. Similar stressors are also often reported by coaches when discussing their concerns over the athlete returning to sport, with the risk of re-injury frequently cited as the biggest concern. These stressors can be placed in three categories:

- **physical stressors** – including the risk of re-injury, the athlete being able to regain match fitness and the athlete making technical adjustments to compensate for the injury

- **social stressors** – including the athlete feeling isolated from the team, an increased sense of pressure from significant others to return to sport and being beaten by people that they used to beat prior to the injury (negative social comparisons)

- **performance stressors** – including the athlete falling behind others in their progress, losing/regaining their place in the squad or team and being able to reach pre-injury performance levels.

As a sports therapist, you play a central role in helping the athlete return to sport after injury. The following recommendations help to ease the athlete's transition back to sport.

- Establish realistic expectations.
- Use appropriate goal setting techniques.
- Use psychological skills and counselling to help the athlete rebuild their confidence.

- Allow athletes to return to sport when they are ready rather than forcing them to return early.

- Facilitate contact with athletes who have had similar injuries and experiences.

- Establish the athlete's motivation to return to sport.

- Keep athletes involved with the sport/team where possible during the injury period.

- Allow extra one-to-one training time.

- Foster social support.

Client dependency

An issue that can occur in therapy settings is that of client dependency. Dependency could manifest itself in the following ways:

- the client struggling to cope as the number of sessions with the therapist is reduced

- the client making repeated attempts to contact the therapist outside of scheduled sessions

- a client asks for support which is outside the scope of a sports therapist.

One method of dealing with dependency is to discuss with the client why they feel they need support from the therapist and to highlight the positive elements of finishing the rehabilitation programme, e.g. it is a sign they are able to return to competitive sport. You should also make use of your referral network to support the client. For instance, if a client exhibits signs of substance misuse or suicidal thoughts you must refer them to a more appropriate professional. When dealing with dependency issues, you must stay within the limitations of practice. You cannot solve every issue your client may have.

Case study

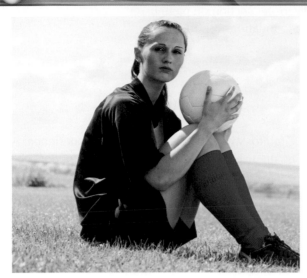

Louise is representing her youth international football team and is in her second year at college. There is a major youth international tournament coming up and there has just been a change of coaching set-up in the team where a new manager and set of coaches have come in. Currently, Louise's father is suffering from testicular

cancer and is in the early stages of treatment. Louise would normally be able talk to her partner about this but they have recently split up and this is playing on Louise's mind. Louise has started to worry a lot about how she is playing and training – and has started to worry that she may lose her place in the national team. During a game for her national team, Louise picks up an injury which means that she is going to be sidelined until one month before the tournament starts.

1. What are the different stressors and injury risk factors associated with this case?

2. What will some of Louise's responses to the injury be?

3. How could a sports therapist help Louise in this instance?

4. Would referrals to any other professionals be appropriate in this case?

5. How do you think Louise is going to react on her estimated return to sport, given how close it is to the international tournament?

Check your understanding

1. How does the stress injury model of sports injury try to explain the causes of sports injury?

2. How can the attitudes of significant others increase the risk of sports injury?

3. What are the different models of responses to sports injury and how do they try to explain the psychological responses of injured athletes?

4. What signs should a sports therapist look for as indicators of poor adjustment to injury?

5. What are the typical behaviours of athletes who are adjusting to injury well and adhering to their programme correctly?

6. According to Heil (1993), what are the different stages in the rehabilitation of clients?

7. Why is social support a key factor in sports injury?

8. What does the acronym 'SMARTS' stand for and why is it important?

9. What are the benefits of using psychological skills training with injured athletes?

10. What are the different techniques used with injured athletes to aid rehabilitation?

To obtain answers to these questions visit the companion website at www.pearsonfe.co.uk/foundationsinsport

Useful resources

To obtain a secure link to the websites below, see the Websites section on page ii or visit the companion website at www.pearsonfe.co.uk/foundationsinsport.

Association for Applied Sport Psychology

Institute of Sports Psychology

Athletic Insight – the online journal of psychology

Further reading

Bianco, T., and Eklund, R.C. (2001). Conceptual considerations for social support research in sport and exercise settings: The case of sport injury. *Journal of sport and exercise psychology*, Vol. 23, 85–107.

Brewer, B.W. (1994). Review and critique of models of psychological adjustment to sports injury. *Journal of applied sport psychology*, Vol. 6, 87–100.

Brewer, B.W. (1998). Adherence to sport injury rehabilitation programs. *Journal of applied sport psychology*, Vol. 10, 70–82.

Carson, F., and Polman, R.C.J. (2010). The facilitative nature of avoidance coping within sports injury rehabilitation. *Scandinavian journal of medicine and science in sports*, Vol. 20, 235–240.

Cohen, R., Nordin, S.M., Abrahamson, E. (2010). Psychology and sport rehabilitation. In P. Comfort and E. Abrahamson (eds.). *Sports injury rehabilitation and injury prevention*. Chichester: Wiley-Blackwell, 275–296.

Crossman, J. (ed.) (2001). *Coping with sports injuries: Psychological strategies for rehabilitation*. Oxford: Oxford University Press.

Cupal, D.D., and Brewr, B.W. (2001). Effects of relaxation imagery on knee strength, reinjury anxiety, and pain following anterior cruciate ligament reconstruction. *Rehabilitation psychology*, Vol. 46, 28–43.

Dreidiger, M., Hall, C. and Callow, N. (2006). Imagery use by injured athletes: A qualitative study. *Journal of sports sciences*, Vol. 24, 61–271.

Granito, V.J. (2001). Athletic injury experience: A qualitative focus group approach. *Journal of sport behaviour*, Vol. 24, 62–82.

Heil, J. (ed.) (1993). *Psychology of sports injury*. Champaign: Human Kinetics.

Ievleva, L., and Orlick, T. (1991). Mental links to enhanced healing: An exploratory study. *The sport psychologist*, Vol. 5, 25–40.

Ivarsson, A. and Johnson, U. (2010). Psychological factors as predictors of injuries among senior soccer players. A prospective study. *Journal of medicine and science in sports,* Vol. 20, 235–240.

Johnson, U., and Ivarsson, A. (2011). Psychological predictors of injury amongst junior soccer players. *Scandinavian journal of medicine and science in sports*, Vol. 21, 129–136.

Kolt, G., and Kirby, R. (1996). Injury in Australian competitive female gymnasts: A psychological perspective. *Australian physiotherapy*, Vol. 42, 121–126.

Kornspan, A.S. (2009). *Fundamentals of sport and exercise psychology*. Champaign: Human Kinetics.

Kübler-Ross, E. (1969). *On Death and Dying*. New York: Macmillan.

O'Connor, E., Heil, J., Harmer, P., and Zimmerman, I. (2005). Injury. In J. Taylor and G. Wilson (eds.). *Applying sport psychology: Four perspectives*. Champaign: Human Kinetics, pp. 187–206.

Pargman, D. (ed.) (2007). *Psychological bases of sports injuries*. Morgantown: Fitness Information Technology.

Patterson, E.L., Smith, R.E., and Everett, J.J. (1998). Psychosocial factors as predictors of ballet injuries: Interactive effects of life stress and social support. *Journal of sport behaviour*, Vol. 21, 101–112.

Petitpas, A. and Danish, M. (1995). Caring for injured athletes. In S.M. Murphy (ed.) Sport Psychology Interventions, Champaign: Human Kinetics, 225–281.

Petrie, T.A. (1993). Coping skills, competitive trait anxiety and playing status: moderating effects on the life – stress injury relationship. *Journal of sport and exercise psychology*, Vol. 15, 261–274.

Podlog, L. and Eklund, R.C. (2005). Return to sport after a serious injury: A retrospective examination of motivation and outcomes. *Journal of sport rehabilitation*, Vol. 14, 20–34.

Podlog, L., and Eklund, R.C. (2007). The psychosocial aspects of a return to sport following serious injury: A review of literature from a self – determination perspective. *Psychology of sport and exercise*, Vol. 8, 535–566.

Scherzer, C.M., & Williams, J.M. (2008). Bringing sport psychology into the athletic training room. *Athletic therapy today*, Vol. 13, 15–17.

Smith H.W. (1994). *The 10 natural laws of successful time and life management: Proven strategies for increased productivity and inner peace*. New York: Warner.

Steffen, K.; Pensgaard, A. M.; Bahr, R. (2009). Self-reported psychological characteristics as risk factors for injuries in female youth football. *Scandinavian journal of medicine and science in sports*, Vol. 19, 442–451.

Taylor, J. and Taylor, S. (1997). *Psychological approaches to sports injury rehabilitation*. Gathersburg, MD: Aspen.

Udry, E. (1996). Social support: Exploring its role in the context of athletic injuries. *Journal of sport rehabilitation*, Vol. 5, 151–163.

Udry, E., Gould, D., Bridges, D., and Beck, L. (1997). Down but not out: Athlete responses to season-ending ski injuries. *Journal of sport and exercise psychology*, Vol. 3, 229–248

Walker, N., Thatcher, J., and Lavalee, D. (2007). Psychological responses to injury in competitive sport: A critical review. *The journal of the royal society for the promotion of health*, Vol. 127, 174–180.

Weinberg, R.S. and Gould, D. (2007). *Foundations of sport and exercise psychology*, 4th Edition. Champaign: Human Kinetics.

Wiese-Bjornstal, D.M., Smith, A.M., Shaffer, S.M. and Marrey, M.A. (1998). An integrated model of response to sports injury: Psychological and sociological dynamics. *Journal of applied sport psychology*, Vol. 10, 46–69.

Williams, J.M. and Andersen, M.B. (1998). Psychosocial antecedents of sports injury: Review and critique of the stress and injury model. *Journal of applied sport psychology*, Vol. 10, 5–25.

Williams, J.M. and Andersen, M.B. (2007). Psychosocial antecedents of sports injury and interventions for risk reduction. In G. Tenebaum & R.C. Eklund (eds). Handbook of Research in Sport Psychology, 3rd Edition, Hoboken: John Wiley and Sons. 379–403.

Williams, J.M. and Scherzer, C.B. (2010). Injury Risk and Rehabilitation. In J.M. Williams (ed.) *Applied Sport Psychology: Personal Growth to Peak Performance*. Boston: McGraw-Hill, 379–403.

Williams, J.M., and Roepke, N. (1993). Psychology of injury and injury rehabilitation. In Singer, R.N., Murphey, M., & Tennant, K.L. *Handbook of Sport Psychology*, Macmillan, New York, 815–839.

Chapter 12

Ethics and safety

Introduction

A professional therapist will always work within their own scope of practice, using only those techniques or knowledge and understanding in which they have been fully trained and assessed. A safe therapist is one who keeps up-to-date with their skills and is always aware of changes or developments within their profession. This can be done by attending practical updating workshops, seminars or courses, reading peer-reviewed journals or even by reflecting on their own practice – very often it will be a combination of all of them.

Safety is a primary consideration in every aspect of a sports therapist's work, whether this is working as an employee or self-employed. It is your responsibility to work safely and professionally at all times.

Learning outcomes

After you have read this chapter you should be able to:

- identify the health and safety legislation that the therapist should be aware of

- discuss the importance of working safely

- demonstrate a risk analysis for different sports and therapy environments

- identify aspects of professional conduct

- explain ethical considerations when working as a therapist.

Health and safety legislation

Legislation in the UK and the European Union is complex and constantly changing. You are expected to have up-to-date knowledge of the law and it is your responsibility to be able to put legislation into practice when working. Below are just *some* of the different types of legislation that govern your work. There is other legislation, equally as important, and you should research and keep up-to-date with these changes on a regular basis.

Starting block

Think about some of the safety issues you would have to consider when working with teams and individuals.

- What safety precautions would you have to consider?
- Are there any regulations you should be aware of?
- What ethical considerations should you consider when working?

Table 12.1: Some of the legislation that affects a therapist's working practice

Legislation	Description	How it relates to a sports therapy practice
Health and Safety at Work etc. Act (1974)	Safe working practices along with regulations Employers must take responsibility for the health and safety of anyone who enters their premises	Safe working environment relating to equipment, systems of training and work, personal protection, health and safety of clients, colleagues and any visitors
Management of Health and Safety at Work Regulations (1999)	Provision for minimising risks and hazards; procedures for emergency situations ; ensuring there are competent and trained staff to undertake risk assessments	May include training all staff to ensure that risks and hazards are identified, and planning what to do in emergency situations particularly when working with a variety of therapists and clients
Employers' Liability (Compulsory Insurance) Act (1969)	Compulsory insurance – employers have a minimum level of 'cover' if an employee becomes ill as a result of their work	Safe working environment and appropriate training for any specialised equipment
Data Protection Act (1998)	The protection of personal data and how such information must be recorded, stored and accessed (both written and electronic versions)	The safe and accurate recording and storage of clients' personal information and treatment records (in a locked fireproof cabinet only accessible by relevant therapists)
The Health and Safety (Display Screen Equipment) Regulations (1992)	Staff who use a display screen are entitled to regular breaks or changes of activity (employers are also responsible for the payment of eye tests for such staff)	May include a receptionist in a practice as well as the therapists who use a computer for work purposes
Fire Precautions Act (1971, 1997 and 1999)	When more than ten people are employed on one floor level, a fire certificate is required. All workplace premises to have up-to-date fire fighting equipment, a fire escape route and marked fire exits Amendments to these regulations (1997 and 1999) – staff should be fully aware and trained in safe fire evacuation The fitting of smoke alarms, fire doors and fire risk assessments must also be undertaken	May include premises such as leisure centres and gyms as well as clinical environments Identify the fire exits and note the meeting place should there be a fire evacuation. The appointment book and visitors' book should include the names of any clients or visitors should there be an emergency – this can be checked against the number of evacuees

Legislation	Description	How it relates to a sports therapy practice
Reporting of Injuries, Disease and Dangerous Occurrences Regulations (RIDDOR) (1995)	Certain diseases and infections must be reported by law if sustained at work. This also includes: • anyone sent to hospital from the workplace • death • a stay of more than 24 hours in hospital • major injury • an inability to work for more than three days	Relevant if there is an accident or an allergy to a product causing anaphylactic shock Injuries may also include concussion, loss of any limbs or digits or those incurred directly as a result of the workplace
Control of Substances Hazardous to Health (COSHH) (2002)	Focuses on exposure to products that may be used in normal practice and that are potentially hazardous	Can include nut-based products that are found in oils, tapes and spray used to improve adherence of tape; hand washing products or even protective gloves that contain latex
Electricity at Work Regulations (1989)	Use, maintenance and installation of electrical equipment (records of electrical testing should be maintained for each piece of equipment)	Equipment such as ultrasound machines, heat lamps, mechanical massage equipment and TENs machines should be regularly maintained in the working environment
Manual Handling Operations Regulations (1992)	Safe techniques to be used when moving, lifting, carrying, pushing or pulling items	May include moving clients or moving/adjusting the treatment plinth, or even reaching up to shelves for new stock
Workplace (Health Safety and Welfare) Regulations (1992)	Concerned with the health and safety of the actual workplace, e.g. toilet and hand washing facilities, supply of drinking water; general cleanliness, working temperature, ventilation, resting facilities	For the therapy practice this includes adequate toilet and hand washing facilities, clean laundry and equipment cleansed appropriately after each client

Note that, if there are more than five employees in a practice, the employer must have a health and safety policy that is accessible to all staff.

Activity

Check to see if there are any local bye-laws that may affect your work. (This may vary from one local authority to another and usually will be in relation to therapists who use sharps such as acupuncture needles.) Indicate which pieces of information must be displayed when in the workplace or sporting environment.

Finally, carry out some research into:

• Employers' Liability (Compulsory Insurance) Act (1969)

• Public liability insurance and professional indemnity insurance.

Remember

Fire exits and doors must never be blocked and should always be easily accessed in case of a fire.

The importance of working safely

You may work in different surroundings such as leisure centres, first aid rooms, specialised clinics, or even pitch side. There will be many different hazards to consider. You should prepare a risk analysis and action plan to address any potential problems or risks that may cause accidents *before* they could happen. Forward planning is a key requirement of working safely and may be a compulsory aspect of maintaining your professional body membership.

As well as considering the health and safety of others, you also need to ensure your own well-being when working, regardless of the environment. Simple steps like good personal hygiene and wearing appropriate clothing and footwear mean you can work at your very best while supporting your different clients.

Table 12.2: Example of a risk analysis record

Stage 1: Identify	Stage 2: Decide	Stage 3: Evaluate	Stage 4: Record	Stage 5: Review	
Identify potential hazards	Who could be harmed and how?	What are you already doing?	Is there any further action needed?	Action by whom?	Date actioned
Specialist tape Spray adhesive	Client and therapist Allergic reaction Anaphylactic shock Localised allergic skin reaction	Conduct a small skin test 24 hours prior to application and record on client's record card Therapist to wear protective gloves when applying spray	Therapist to check client's skin reaction to the test before applying adhesive and tape	Therapist to note on record card date of skin test and actual results of the test	

Risk analysis

Risk analysis, also called risk assessment, is a good way of trying to minimise risks and preventing accidents or injuries. It does not have to be completed by an expert in health and safety. The overall aims are to assess and then control the risks. Risk analysis is usually completed in five stages:

1. Identify any potential hazards – in a sport setting this can be specialised equipment, flooring, products, etc. If you are working in a team then it is helpful if everyone considers potential hazards and risks and takes responsibility towards developing and maintaining safe working practice.

2. Decide who could be harmed and how (including any other people and visitors).

3. Evaluate the risks and decide on any necessary precautions – this may be as basic as recording if they are high, medium or low risk. It may be that some simple changes need to be made, for example providing protective clothing or changing products.

4. Record the findings and implement changes, developing a simple chart and reminding all team members of actions that are taken. The Health and Safety Executive produces a good example of a table that may be used.

5. Review the assessment and update regularly, ideally every year, and particularly if there is a frequency of accidents. A simple amendment to practice can overcome some problems.

You can work safely by liaising with colleagues or holding regular team meetings which have minutes and action plans to record how things may be improved. Clear communication via discussions, notice boards, posters or whiteboards can help to promote a safe working environment. Ideally, everyone should share responsibility for safe practice in all aspects of work. Clearly designated areas for first aid boxes, cin bins (for clinical wastes and disposal of sharps), accident sheets/book, along with regular first aid drills and practice, will help to maintain good standards for the benefit of all.

Activity

Complete a five stage risk assessment of a clinical area and a sports changing room/ shower area.

Activity

Consider the different types of clothing and equipment you would need to ensure your own health and safety when working in the following situations:
- at the touchline and running on to a muddy football pitch during the winter months
- indoors in a small air conditioned clinic
- outdoors in the summer months at a cricket match.

Hazards

You must always look for any potential hazards before you start work. It is everyone's responsibility to contribute to a safe working environment and this includes all employees.

Tripping hazards such as trailing flexes or wires from equipment or computers can easily cause accidents. In changing areas, especially when there are groups of athletes, tripping hazards can include kit bags, clothes or boots left lying on the floor. At the court or pitch side this may be spare equipment, water bottles or even other people such as coaches or touchline judges.

Accidents such as slipping can easily occur when products such as oil or water are splashed on the floor. In showers or hydrotherapy areas, specialist tiles and non-slip flooring are essential to minimise the risk of accident and injury. Spillages should be wiped away immediately and a plastic yellow alert sign indicating a wet floor should be left in place until the surface is dry.

 Remember

A first aid kit should be provided in working areas though the contents may vary slightly in different working environments.

Manual handling

When reaching up or moving heavy items, make sure that appropriate equipment such as stable stepladders or a trolley with wheels is available. Sometimes you may also have to move an individual; if possible, call for help and remember basic first aid principles when you are moving the casualty.

Electrical equipment

All equipment should be regularly checked to make sure that it is fit for purpose and does not need replacing. Electrical equipment should always be well maintained and regularly serviced by a qualified electrician. Some equipment, such as ultrasound machines, may have to be sent away for specialist repairs or servicing and may require you to keep a log of the hours the equipment has been used for. Each piece of equipment should have its own record to indicate that it has been electrically tested; ideally this should be dated and signed by the electrician.

The Electricity at Work Regulations (1989)
require that any electrical equipment that could cause injury is safely maintained. However, the regulations do not specify what needs to be done or who must do the checks. The Health and Safety Executive provides free information to download.

 Key terms

Manual handling – when the body moves, usually lifting items, but it also includes pulling, twisting, pushing or climbing

The Electricity at Work Regulations 1989 – also commonly known as portable appliance testing (PAT)

 Remember

Clients should never be left unsupervised during a treatment, especially if it involves equipment that is connected to any form of power supply.

Chemicals

As part of your work, you and your clients may come into contact with chemicals, some of which can be hazardous. These can include products such as massage preparations (oils, creams and milk), dressings, different types of tape or support materials (zinc oxide, elastic adhesive bandage (EAB) and sticking plasters), or even cleaning products that are used on a daily basis. Ideally, if you need to wear protective gloves, these should be latex free because some clients may also have an allergy to latex.

Employers are required under the Control of Substances Hazardous to Health Regulations (COSHH, 2002) to identify all the products which are used in the working environment that could be potentially hazardous. From this there should then be a written assessment of the likely exposure, and how this may affect employees, clients or any visitors. This regulation helps to promote a safe environment for all parties. However, only those products that are considered to cause harm to the body are recognised as hazardous.
This usually includes any product that:

- comes into contact or can be absorbed though the skin or the eyes (this can also include indirect contact with items such as clothing or working surfaces)

- may enter the body via cuts, abrasions or broken skin
- is inhaled from the working environment
- is ingested via contaminated food or drinks or even via dirty hands
- is injected.

COSSH (2002) allows the employer to draw up a list which can help to determine:

- the products to be used
- who may be exposed to the product, along with times and frequency of exposure
- what actions can be taken to adequately control any exposure.

These action points or remedies can be quite straightforward and may include providing personal protective equipment (PPE), the safe storage and labelling of products, containers being resealed after use, or even ensuring there is appropriate ventilation.

> ### Top tip
>
> Before applying any product to the client, always check they do not have any allergies to it or any of its ingredients and that they are not contraindicated to the treatment.

Infection control

Transmission of infection also needs to be carefully controlled. Coughs, colds, viral infections such as veruccas or fungal infections such as athlete's foot can be easily transmitted from one person to another, especially in communal areas. In sporting environments, clients may share clothing or equipment and so the incidence of cross-infection can often be higher.

You should always thoroughly wash your hands before and after every treatment. Using alcohol-based sanitising gel or foam can also help to reduce the risks of cross-infection (although this is not a substitute for proper hand washing). Where possible, disposable products such as paper towels should be used rather than cloth towels as these can

harbour bacteria. Non-contaminated waste should be thrown away into a lined pedal bin that should have a lid, and this should be emptied at the end of each day or once it becomes full.

> ### Activity
>
> Look at ten products that a therapist may use in their work. Identify the ingredients and indicate how exposure to these products can be controlled. Include any action points that can help to remedy the exposure.

Professional conduct

Codes of professional conduct are a set of minimum standards. They are frequently linked to membership of a professional body or even a national governing body (NGB) in sport. These codes often include student members too. They are usually linked to different behaviours and standards and involve responsibilities, not just for the treatment of clients, but for other people with whom you may come into contact including referees, umpires, spectators and the general public.

Professional conduct usually relates to:

- always acting in the best interest of the client
- ensuring confidentiality of clients' personal information and treatments
- keeping accurate and detailed record cards of treatments
- obtaining informed consent (excluding emergencies)
- acting with honesty and integrity
- declaring any conflicts of interest to relevant parties as and when different situations arise
- always working within your scope of practice – referring on to other professionals when necessary
- continually keeping up-to-date with all aspects of professional development.

In practice you must ensure that you follow the codes that are linked to your professional body. It is not unusual for members (including student members) to have to inform their professional organisation if there are any details that have changed from their initial membership application.

This can include notifying them if you have received:

- any convictions – including any conditional discharges or police cautions relating to any matter but also if that involves:

    - child pornography

    - prison sentences

    - violent acts

    - illegal supplying of drugs

    - charges of dishonesty

- a suspension from duties in any capacity (whether paid or voluntary) particularly if this relates to actual competence and practice as a therapist.

Your own health is also a matter of importance where codes of conduct and practice are concerned. Should there be any significant changes to your health, or you feel that your judgement has become impaired in any way, you should seek professional advice from an appropriate approved medical practitioner or guidance from your professional body. It is important that you provide a confidential explanation because the outcomes may mean that you have to amend your methods of practising or stop altogether in some circumstances.

Remember

A certificate of attendance does not mean that a therapist is competent to practise a particular skill on clients. Usually some method of recorded formal hours of attendance, along with assessment, will need to be undertaken in order for a therapist to be deemed competent.

Liaising with other professionals

You may liaise regularly with other professionals and you may also work with other members of the multidisciplinary team (MDT). However, there could be circumstances when you need to refer a client on to another health care professional for specific assessment, treatment or advice. In these instances you should follow clear procedures so that you act in the best interests of all concerned.

All information relating to any client is confidential and should not be discussed with any other third party without the client's express permission. This is particularly important in relation to an individual's treatment record card which will hold detailed personal information. You must gain written permission from the client on every occasion when information needs to be passed on to another healthcare professional. It is your responsibility to liaise with the client and explain why it is recommended that specific information is shared before gaining their consent; for example, you may wish to refer your client on to a podiatrist because they have repeated foot problems that are not improving. You should never try to indicate what another healthcare professional may say or do – instead you should ask them to seek the advice of this other professional, and then they can decide how to progress matters. Informed decision making is an important aspect of everyone's well-being, and sometimes they may choose not to follow your advice, or even decide that they prefer to wait before acting on such advice.

Professional etiquette is important and you should take care to be discreet and professional at all times, especially when confidential matters are being addressed. Always be thoughtful and respectful and listen carefully to what others are saying. It is unprofessional to criticise or apportion blame to other therapists or colleagues and very often there may be many different perspectives that you are not fully aware of.

You should add a written record on the treatment card to indicate that a referral to another healthcare professional is recommended. Some clients may wish to approach their own healthcare professional and may request that you share any relevant information with them; alternatively other professionals may write to you and ask for specific information relating to a client. In both circumstances you must always gain written consent from the client, ideally a signed letter which is dated and clearly states the name and address of the person to whom the information should be released – this is known as a consent form. Any information that you share should be in a written format to avoid any unclear communication. This should be read and agreed with the client before sending.

If, during a consultation, you establish that a client is contraindicated to a treatment, ask them to visit their GP. They can then check with their doctor if it is safe for the specified treatment to be provided. If the GP agrees, they may provide a brief letter or note to indicate that it is safe to proceed with treatment; very often this is given at the time of the appointment. Before any treatment commences, ask to see the GP's original letter or written consent, and then photocopy and attach it to the client's record card (the original should be returned to the client). All these procedures should be followed before any treatment takes place for contraindicated clients; this is not only for the well-being and safety of the client, but also because your professional indemnity insurance may be cancelled if a claim is made against you for unsafe practice.

Client confidentiality

It is essential that written or computer records are kept secure from all parties except the therapist and the client. You should start from the proposition that these are the only people who should see or access those records. Records should be written in permanent ink – ideally black and, in the case of a written error, correction fluid should never be used, instead a line should be placed though the error and initialled and dated by the therapist, with the correction above the error. Adequate security of all clients' records and their personal data should always be in place.

It is unprofessional, unethical and a breach of client confidentiality to discuss any aspect of your client's care without their express permission. Any images that you take of your client must be taken with their permission and you should not share these without their consent.

Working with children

A sports therapist may not treat anyone under the age of 18 without written consent from a parent or guardian. If a sports therapist works regularly with people under the age of 18 they will be asked to apply for an enhanced Criminal Records Bureau Disclosure (CRB) disclosure. The CRB is an executive agency of the Home Office to help organisations make safer recruitment decisions.

Remember

Clients may not always follow therapist's advice and they always have the right to seek other opinions.

Ethical matters

Ethical matters are linked to a philosophical approach and include the systematic study of morals. Put simply, these are guides for individuals and their personal and professional conduct. It must be remembered that these guides are not universal and may differ between professional bodies according to their codes of practice and professional responsibilities. However, ethics are also about *every* individual considering and acting accordingly in matters of:

- right and wrong
- good and bad
- fairness
- justice and virtue
- morality.

Professional bodies or national governing bodies (NGBs) often provide guidance relating to ethical issues or matters. However, you have an individual responsibility to make sure that you always act and perform with professionalism and integrity, even when other people may be unhappy with your decision. This may be evident in sports when other people try to coerce a team or any of its members to behave irresponsibly, even when that behaviour does not inflict personal harm on others. Behaving appropriately and doing the 'right thing' is about working to professional and ethical or moral standards. They should be followed regardless of whether an individual or team wins or loses a game, or a client is pressured into returning to sport before they are fully fit.

Key term

Code of ethics – a set of professional behaviours or a set of formal rules and regulations often linked to a professional body

Beauchamp and Childress (2001) have produced a widely used framework that you could use as a general guide. However, each category leaves you to consider each individual situation and the associated circumstances.

- **Respect for autonomy:** respecting the decision-making capacities of autonomous persons; enabling individuals to make reasoned, informed choices.

- **Beneficence:** this considers the balancing of benefits of treatment against the risks and costs; the healthcare professional should act in a way that benefits the patient.

- **Non malfeasance:** avoiding the causation of harm; the healthcare professional should not harm the patient. All treatment involves some harm, even if minimal, but the harm should not be disproportionate to the benefits of treatment.

- **Justice:** distributing benefits, risks and costs fairly; the notion that patients in similar positions should be treated in a similar manner.

Informed consent

All therapists should gain consent from their clients after the subjective and objective assessment and before commencing any treatment. You should fully explain to them:

- the proposed treatment or interventions as a result of the objective findings

- why the treatment(s) may be of benefit to them and the realistic results of the treatments

- how the treatments may feel during the process, e.g. warm, cool

- the likely results that may be experienced after the treatment, e.g. discomfort, increased movement, reduction of pain

- the frequency and duration of treatments and the likely outcomes of each session

- what the client can do to help support their treatment during and in between therapy sessions

- they must ask questions they would like answering in relation to the proposed treatment.

If the client is satisfied with the explanations, and agrees to the treatment, they are giving informed *consent* to progress with the planned interventions. They can decide to stop receiving treatment at any time (even if it is not always in their best interest), although you should try to discuss why they would like to cease treatment. It is good practice to formally write on a client's record card the reason why they are stopping treatment.

You also have professional responsibility to constantly review the treatment and you should be prepared to amend, cease or refer on to another appropriate healthcare professional if the treatment(s) is/are ineffective and not benefitting the client. Reviewing the treatments after each session and in between visits can help to establish whether the interventions are appropriate and relevant.

Activity

Compile a list of different reasons why a client may wish to stop receiving treatment. How could you solve some of these issues for the client?

Case study

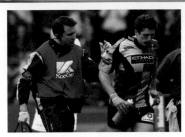

Carry out some research into the 2009 quarter finals of the Heineken Cup match when the English rugby union team Harlequins played Leicester.

A controversial incident took place involving a player faking an injury which resulted in a ban. Once you have completed your research consider the following questions.

1. How would you manage a situation if you were asked by a team member to remove a non-injured client from the pitch with a 'fake injury'?

2. As a practising therapist for an amateur local sports team, how can you ensure confidentiality of client's records?

3. Which members of the team would you share a client's record card information with?

4. If another member of the MDT asked you if a client is fit to compete in a local game, how would you respond?

5. A client has been receiving treatment for 2 months and is not satisfied with their therapist's advice about returning to training and competing in their chosen sport. They ask you for advice on their treatment. What would you do?

Check your understanding

1. Name three pieces of legislation that are concerned with health and safety.

2. Which legislation is important in the storing and retrieval of client's record cards?

3. Name four different environments that a therapist may work in.

4. Why is it important that a therapist maintains good personal hygiene?

5. Name three different types of hazards that a therapist may experience in a clinical environment.

6. State three ways in which products may cause harm and enter the body.

7. What does informed consent mean?

8. State four pieces of information that the therapist must include in order to work towards achieving informed consent.

9. What is a code of ethics?

10. When would a therapist need to tell their professional body about changes in their circumstances?

To obtain answers to these questions visit the companion website at www.pearsonfe.co.uk/foundationsinsport

Useful resources

To obtain a secure link to the websites below, see the Websites section on page ii or visit the companion website at www.pearsonfe.co.uk/foundationsinsport.

Maintaining portable and transportable electrical equipment – a publication from the HSE

Five steps to risk assessment – a leaflet from the HSE

Hand washing advice for patients and visitors – advice from BRH University Hospitals NHS Trust

Criminal Records Bureau checks

Further reading

Anderson, M.K., Parr, G.P. and Hall, S.J. (2009). *Foundations of Athletic Training* 4th Edition. Philadelphia: Lippincott, Williams & Wilkins.

Beauchamp, T. and Childress, J. (2001). *Principles of Biomedical Ethics* 5th Edition. Open University Press.

Comfort, P. and Abrahamson, E. (2010). *Sports Rehabilitation and Injury Prevention*. Chichester: Wiley Blackwell.

Morgan, W.J., Meier, K.V. and Schneider, A.J., (2001). *Ethics in Sport*. Champaign: Human Kinetics.

Ward, K. (2004). *Hands on Sports Therapy*. London: Thomson Learning.

Chapter 13

Planning and practice

Introduction

Success in sports therapy is linked to your ability to relate to the caring aspect of the profession, and complying with industry professional standards. Good first impressions are vital.

Industry professional standards must be met, requiring all graduate and postgraduate therapists to continually drive professional standards forward. Sports therapists need to be protected from unwanted claims, and clients should receive treatment from fully qualified sports therapists. The title 'sports therapist' is not a protected title and thus anyone can trade, and treat clients, under the name. Many therapists who are inadequately qualified, not insured and have no affiliation to a regulatory body work under the title of sports therapist. Do not let this happen to you.

This chapter will develop your knowledge of sports therapy planning and practice. Professional practice will consolidate the benchmark standard for qualifications, insurance, regulatory affiliation, your fitness to practise and medical liaison; professional planning will facilitate your planning of equipment, setting up a treatment room and the consultation process.

Learning outcomes

After you have read this chapter you should be able to:

- explain professional practice within the industry
- describe the types of insurance a sports therapist may need
- identify and describe the equipment a sports therapist will require
- discuss professional practice in relation to the consultation process.

Starting block

As a sport therapist you may need to refer patients to other practitioners or medical personnel.

- List the healthcare professionals that you may need to liaise with. For each one, think why you may need to refer a client to them. What services can they offer that you can't?

Professional practice within the industry

First impressions

It takes approximately 5–10 seconds for a person to evaluate you upon first meeting. The opinion they form of you is principally based on your appearance, body language, demeanour, mannerisms and dress. The first impression sets the standard and, if you give the wrong one, the chances of reversing it are unlikely.

Figure 13.1: First impressions are formed within the first 10 seconds. How can you ensure you make a good impression?

While you are an individual with your own identity, you have to conform to the industry you are entering. You are working within the service industry, the public are your clients and are paying for your services and expertise – they expect certain standards from you. Just as a business person would dress in business attire, and a nurse, member of the police or fire brigade would wear a uniform, you are expected to dress appropriately.

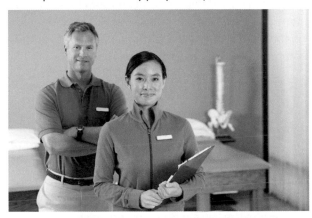

Figure 13.2: What other factors should you consider about your personal appearance?

Stop and think

Think of a professional you have visited. What was your first impression and why?

Spending time preparing yourself, the treatment room and the work you are going to do will help to create a good impression. Bear in mind the following.

- Prepare yourself mentally – be calm and relaxed.
- Ensure your clothes are clean, ironed and appropriate.
- Arrive early so you can organise your day ahead.
- Do not wear jewellery.
- Keep your nails short and do not wear nail varnish.
- Cover cuts or wounds.
- Do not attend work with an infectious disease, or spread germs from colds and flu.
- Wear subtle make-up and ensure your hair is tidy and off your face. Long hair should always be tied back.

Building a rapport

Building a rapport with your client is essential to earn their trust and loyalty. Show respect with an appropriate attitude; be polite and sensitive, and address your client appropriately. Do not assume first name terms. Ask your client how they wish to be addressed. For example, you could refer to your client as Mr Cox or Mrs Cox or Ms Cox although most clients will request you call them by their first name. Speak formally, especially with new clients. *Chapter 15: Work-based learning* will further address communication skills and body language.

Fit for sports therapy?

The role of a sports therapist can be physically demanding. It's important to maintain your own fitness, flexibility and good posture to prevent aches, pains and repetitive strain injury (RSI) – and to carry out your duties effectively while presenting a professional image.

Case study

You are running pitch side for a semi-professional football team. At 80 minutes a player pulls up on the pitch clutching his left hamstring. He is on the opposite side to the pitch to where you are situated. Henry has been receiving treatment on the left hamstring for the past three weeks.

1. How quickly can you reach the player on the opposite side of the pitch?

2. Is it possible for you to reduce your response time by improving your own fitness levels?

While it is not a requirement for a sports therapist to play sport, it is extremely useful if you have a good understanding of a variety of sports. You should understand what the sport involves, technical and tactical aspects, as well as the fitness and training requirements. This will help you understand how injuries arise, **injury aetiology** and the need for return to sports participation as early as is safely possible.

Key term

Injury aetiology – the study of how injury is caused or originates

Sports therapy and the medical hierarchy

Sports therapists are not medically qualified but you need to understand your role within the medical hierarchy. The GP is generally the first person who is presented with any medical complaint. They offer advice, prescribe medication or refer on to a consultant for diagnosis or for further treatment. The approach taken by the GP is dependent upon the severity and nature of the complaint. A sports therapist should always refer a client presenting with any serious health or injury problem to a GP and must never mimic their role. GPs and consultants work closely with physiotherapists – chartered physiotherapists are classified within the medical profession and are registered with the Health Professions Council (HPC).

In the case of an emergency, the nearest hospital accident and emergency department will be your first port of call. As more people understand the role of sports therapists, the working relationship with medical personnel is advancing. The role of a sports therapist is covered fully in *Chapter 15: Work-based learning*.

Remember

If you need to refer a client to another professional, explain the reason for referral and how they could benefit. Do not alarm or frighten the client.

Protected professional titles

Professional titles such as Consultant in Sport and Exercise Medicine, Sports Physician, GP and chartered physiotherapist are protected by the General Medical Council and the Health Professions Council (HPC). The role of the HPC is to protect the public and regulate health professions. Anyone unsuitably qualified is unable to trade or call themselves by these titles by law. You can read more about the HPC on their website (see Useful resources on page 175).

Sports therapy training standard

Sports therapy is not regulated by the HPC. This means that many people are able to call themselves a sports therapist. Industry regulatory bodies are trying to achieve HPC status for sports therapy which is considered a complementary therapy, and which has experienced massive growth over the past 10 years.

The minimum standard for training as a sports therapist is reading for a 3 year Bachelor of Science (BSc) Degree in Sports Therapy. There are a variety of pathways in which to achieve your BSc and one of the most popular routes is to first complete a Foundation Degree in Sports Therapy. Foundation degrees are designed to equip you for a particular area of work, as well as developing your **transferable skills**. They have a high vocational and work experience content. Postgraduate pathways are readily available to a sports therapist including sports rehabilitation, and physiotherapy. If you have a BSc in Sport Science, and wish to train as a sports therapist, then consider undertaking a Masters Degree in Sports Therapy.

 Key term

Transferable skills – general skills that can be used in any type of job

Regulatory bodies

You need to know the main regulatory bodies which are active in the field of sports therapy.

- The Society of Sports Therapists (SST) is actively involved in regulating the industry. Their aims include:
  - improving the standards of sports therapy
  - validating nationally recognised courses
  - monitoring and advising on sports therapy matters.

  For full information about the society, their aims and how to join, go to the Society of Sports Therapists website (see *Useful resources* on page 175).

- The British Association of Sports Rehabilitators and Trainers (BASRaT) represent the sport and exercise-based injury prevention, treatment and rehabilitation industry. BASRaT aims to ensure the highest standard of healthcare for

the physically active. For full information about BASRaT, go to their website (again, see *Useful resources* on page 175).

A sports therapist should be appropriately qualified, i.e. hold BSc (Hons) Sports Therapy or BSc (Hons) Sports Rehabilitation as a minimum, be affiliated to a regulatory body such as SST or BASRaT, and hold valid and appropriate insurances.

Sports therapy versus sports massage

Sports therapy encompasses a portfolio of skills (*Chapter 15: Work-based learning* addresses the skills of a sports therapist), one of which is sports massage. Individuals can choose to train as a sports massage practitioner (which is not sports therapy) via approved weekend, part-time and evening study. The course should be approved by an appropriate awarding body, meet the new national occupational standards for sports massage at the appropriate level (released 2010) and be endorsed by the Sports Massage Association (SMA). Vocational Training Charitable Trust (VTCT) offers a portfolio of courses within the field of sports massage, complementary and holistic therapy. The Sports Massage level 3, 4 and 5 specifications reflect the new national occupational standards and are endorsed by the SMA. Private training providers offer a range of courses which are approved by insurance companies, but not all are reflective of the National Occupation Standards or endorsed or affiliated to regulatory bodies. You should ask before you enrol.

A sports massage practitioner should be appropriately qualified, i.e. VTCT Level 3 Sports Massage as a minimum, ideally Level 4, particularly if you want to work in elite or professional sport. You should be affiliated to a regulatory body such as SMA at the appropriate level, and hold valid and appropriate insurances.

Types of insurance

As a working therapist you must have public liability and professional indemnity insurance. Obtaining the correct insurance demonstrates you have a professional approach to your work. If someone should make a claim against you in the event of an accident in your treatment environment, or have a reason to claim against you, you will have the appropriate insurance cover to address the claim.

- **Public liability** – provides protection from claims made by members of the public or clients who sustain an injury or loss as a result of the business. Even the most conscientious and experienced therapists cannot guarantee a client will not trip over, slip on the ice at the entrance to their clinic or misplace a possession. If a claim for compensation is made, you will be insured, any medical bills will be covered, and losses can be replaced. Public liability insurance does not provide protection for a claim resulting from treatment or advice given.

- **Professional indemnity insurance** – protects you from a claim which may arise from breaches of duty of care, neglect, error, omission or loss of documents/data or unintentional breach of confidence. This provides insurance whether you are treating a client or providing advice.

> **Top tip**
>
> A working therapist should have as a minimum public liability and professional indemnity insurance. Shop around for competitive quotes.

- **Risk equipment and products protection** – protects your business equipment and products against loss or damage – applicable if you rely on expensive equipment and use a wide range of products.

- **Products liability insurance** – protects from any claim (injury or damage) as a result of any defect in goods sold, supplied or demonstrated to the client by the therapist.

- **Employer's liability** – if you have employees it is a legal requirement that you hold employer's liability insurance. It protects the employer from injuries sustained by any employees on the premises.

Insurance policies vary between companies so read them in full and ensure you are covered for all treatments you administer. Most policies offer a standard £1 million cover but this can be extended for a premium. Standard policies generally do not insure you to treat professional sports people. You will be required to provide further details of the professional sports person and seek confirmation from your insurance company before you commence

any treatment. The insurance company will probably charge you for additional insurance cover.

Cover can be obtained from companies such as:

- Independent Professional Therapists International

- Society of Sports Therapists

- Norwich Union

- Federation of Holistic Therapists.

> **Top tip**
>
> It is an insurance requirement that you keep accurate, legible and up-to-date records.

Equipment

Your equipment will depend upon your type of business. If you decide to work as a mobile therapist and/or at a sporting event your equipment must be portable and lightweight. However, if you decide to be clinic based, you can ensure the environment is comfortable and ergonomically friendly. Consider the financial implications of your purchases. There are a number of suppliers of equipment such as Physique and Physiomed. Get competitive quotes and obtain professional advice. The main items of equipment you may purchase include a massage couch, towels, couch roll, massage medium such as oil, talcum powder or cream and hand sanitisation gel.

Massage couch

A lightweight portable couch should:

- be sturdy and strong (be aware of maximum weight limits)

- fold in half with secure catches and have a strong protective case.

It is worth considering purchasing a couch trolley to ease transportation. If you are thinking of buying a permanent fixed couch, consider whether you want a hydraulic or electric operated couch. Your main deciding factor will be determining where the electric power point supply is within the clinic as trailing wires will contravene health and safety.

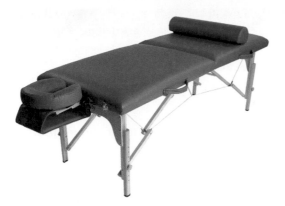

Figure 13.3: What should you consider when purchasing a portable couch?

Towels/couch roll

You will need one large bath sheet, one bath towel and three hand towels as a minimum. The bath sheet and bath towel will be used to maintain the client's modesty and provide warmth, while two hand towels will be used as supports with the third towel rolled into a sausage shape to provide comfort when the head is placed in the face hole.

At an event it is a good idea to take a supply of couch roll to cover the couch which can be disposed of and replaced between clients. This helps to maintain a clean couch as your clients may be perspiring, muddy or wet.

Massage medium

There is a wide range of massage mediums available to the therapist including oils, creams and talcum powder. It is imperative the therapist ensures the client does not have any allergies to any products, particularly those products pre-blended with aromatherapy oils or nut-based oils. More information on massage mediums can be found on page 44, *Chapter 3: Fundamentals of sports massage*.

Ice

Ice is a popular treatment method. If you are based in a clinic you should have access to ice via an ice machine or a freezer. If you are working at an event or running pitch side the weather will have an impact. On cooler days a picnic cooler filled with ice will stay frozen for several hours. Ice can be placed in a plastic bag, tied and applied to the client. On warmer days you could use disposable ice packs which are activated when you break the seal.

Ice massage is popular. You can make your own ice massage sticks by putting some ice in a plastic cup, placing a lolly pop stick in the middle, filling with water and freezing. When you are ready, peel the plastic cup away and use it to massage. You should only use one ice block per client.

Hand sanitisation gel

Hand sanitisation gel is essential if you do not have access to running water. Clean your hands before and after every treatment.

Your treatment room

Treatment rooms can be found in sports clubs, health clubs, leisure centres, complementary therapy clinics and osteopathy clinics, and some therapists convert a room in their house. Wherever you decide to base your room, you should consider the following points.

- Hygiene is vital. The room must be clean, tidy and free from any obstacles. A risk assessment must be completed (see *Chapter 12: Ethics and safety*, page 159).
- Have a first aid kit to hand, and a phone in case of emergency.
- There should be washing facilities in the room or close by.
- The room should have adequate ventilation, and a good source of heating.
- If your room is in a public area, ensure your clients' privacy by having clear signage.

Security

When you consider security, theft or damage springs to mind. However, it includes security of premises, equipment, stock and treatment records, belongings of the therapist and client, your takings and protection of the therapist and client. Security is just as important for a sole trader as it is for an employer – the only difference is the scale of security. Training should be held for employees, and signatures obtained from them to confirm they have received the training and understand their role.

Security issues to consider include:

- installing a burglar alarm and smoke detector, window locks and door locks (preferably a five lever mortice lock conforming to insurance standards)

- ensuring the facility is well lit if therapists have evening appointments

- using a fireproof locked cabinet for the storage of record cards and lockable lockers for therapists' and clients' use

- monitoring stock levels (stock should be kept in a lockable cupboard)

- limiting the amount of money in the till and a safe in a secure place to store any money

- ensuring no therapist ever works on their own.

 Top tip

Clients' possessions are your responsibility. Make sure they are locked away or the client places them in their bag.

The consultation process

A consultation must take place before any treatment commences. Depending on the complexity of the case the consultation will take approximately 30–45 minutes. (Work within the scope of your abilities – if you are unsure at any time, refer the client to another therapist or medical practitioner.) Explain the prospective treatment to your client and gather and document information about them in order to provide a full, safe and effective treatment. At times you will find clients are reluctant to divulge information – stress that all information is confidential, records are stored securely and you are unable to proceed any further without the relevant information.

For details of consultations, refer to *Chapter 2: Introduction to sports injury and assessment*, page 30.

Agreement and confirmation of short-, medium- and long-term goals should be documented. *Chapter 2: Introduction to sports injury and assessment* contains an example of a consultation form (page 30).

 Remember

If you feel your client is behaving inappropriately you do not have to treat them.

SMART goals

Any goal you set for your client or yourself, whether treatment related or in your personal development, should follow the principles of the acronym SMART.

Specific

Measurable

Achievable

Realistic

Timely

- **Specific and measurable** – a goal should be clear. It defines what you want to happen, and will focus your efforts on achieving it. The goal should be measurable so you can document and monitor progress. For example: a short-term goal may be to reduce pain levels from 8 out of 10 to 2 out of 10 within 10 days; a medium-term goal may be to improve knee flexion range of movement from 100° to 130° within 4 weeks; a long-term goal may be to return to full sports participation within 7 weeks. You should consider and document:
  - **what** treatments methods you are going to administer
  - **why** this treatment method is the most appropriate
  - **how** are you going to do this with clinical justification.
- **Achievable and realistic** – the goals must be achievable and realistic. If the goal is to reduce pain levels within 1 day, or to improve knee flexion within 1 day, it may not be achievable or realistic. This can demotivate the client and compromise your professional reputation.
- **Timely** – set a time frame for goal achievement.

Treatment records

Check your insurance policy to determine the exact length of time treatment records must be kept for. On average most policies state that your treatment records should be kept for 6 years, although the recommendation is 7 years. The statute of limitations normally allows 3 years for a claim to be brought against you from the point a problem was discovered. Some insurance companies recommend if you treat children or clients with disabilities (such as a mental illness) you maintain the records indefinitely. This is due to the extended amount of time the courts allow. In some cases there may be no statute of limitation. In the result of any claim your treatment notes are the main source of defence.

Your treatment records should adequately record each treatment given to every client. Records should include full details of the subjective and objective consultation process, treatments administered, treatment result, aftercare and any instructions given to the client. Make sure the records are intelligible to others, fully comprehensive, signed appropriately and stored in a locked, and preferably fireproof, place.

> **Top tip**
>
> **Informed and written consent** is a legal requirement. Forgetting is not an option.

Aftercare

Aftercare should always be given following any treatment. This ensures an effective treatment process. Advice given will differ between clients, although a common theme will be evident among some recommendations. Think about the following topics and if they are applicable to your client for advice:

- immediate common aftercare such as rest, use of ice for 24–48 hours following a deep treatment or as an analgesic effect, drinking water and avoiding alcohol
- stretches to facilitate the elongation of fibres and further increase range of movement
- rehabilitation exercise, for example proprioception, range of movement, strength, endurance or hydrotherapy
- relaxation techniques to help with anxiety, stress or mental focus

- maintenance of good posture, altering working ergonomics
- nutritional advice such as hydration, carbohydrate intake pre- and post-exercise
- the use of thermal therapy and cryotherapy
- modifications to exercise and training schedule
- recommendation of number of treatments and treatment length
- prehabilitation strategies to prevent future injuries.

Aftercare should ideally be provided in a written format, but must always be thoroughly documented in the treatment records.

Evaluating effectiveness of treatments

It is essential that you evaluate the effectiveness of your treatments. To do this, clearly and accurately record subjective and objective information, as well as short-, medium- and long-term goals.

> **Key terms**
>
> **Informed consent** – informing your client by fully explaining the treatments to be administered
>
> **Aftercare** – includes any instruction given to a client to complete after the treatment (ideally in a written format)

Principally you are analysing the information present at the beginning and the end of the treatment process. You will identify any improvements and clinically justify why they are evident. Alternatively, if there is no improvement, identify why the treatment was ineffective, and what alternative treatment methods you could have used, or if you need to refer the client to another practitioner.

Information you could use for your analysis includes:

- client feedback during, after and between treatments with regard to the reported signs and symptoms such as pain levels
- subjective information such as feedback regarding well-being, ease with which activities are completed, reduction in fatigue and improved performance

173

- objective information such as a range of movement and active tests (measured with a **goniometer**), resistive muscle testing (a degree of subjectivity will always be evident due to assessment technique)

- reflection on your short-, medium- and long-term goals.

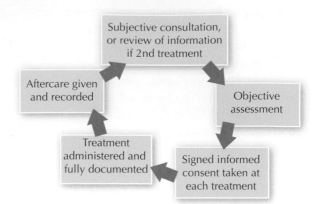

Figure 13.4: The treatment cycle. Why is it important to review the client's notes on their second visit?

Key term

Goniometer – an instrument used to measure the angles of a joint

Case study

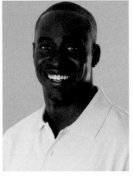

William Gallagher is a self-employed therapist and has worked hard over the past 12 years to attain his position within the industry. He has a portfolio of qualifications including an MSc Sports Therapy, and a vast range of experience. After having his own premises built, and advertising via word of mouth only, the clinic is enjoying a thriving business. Will has a good portfolio of contacts to whom he can refer clients including a physiologist, sports psychologist, sports scientist, strength and condition coach, podiatrist and osteopath. Clients feel fully supported throughout their rehabilitation and during their ongoing prehabilitation. Will has a part-time position available for a suitable candidate for pitch side support. Expenses will be reimbursed but own equipment needs to be sourced.

1. State the qualifications you need to aspire to, to achieve this position.

2. State the regulatory body of which you should become a member.

3. Describe the insurance requirements you need to adhere to as a qualified therapist.

4. Discuss the equipment you will need for your pitch side duties.

Check your understanding

1. Explain why the first impression of the therapist is important.

2. Describe the benchmark industry standards for a sports therapist in terms of qualifications, insurance and regulatory bodies.

3. Describe six security issues you should consider for your treatment room.

4. Describe the key stages of the consultation process.

5. You are attending the Great North Run as a sports therapist to administer pre- and post-event massage. List all the equipment you will need to take with you.

To obtain answers to these questions visit the companion website at www.pearsonfe.co.uk/foundationsinsport

Useful resources

To obtain a secure link to the websites below, see the Websites section on page ii or visit the companion website at www.pearsonfe.co.uk/foundationsinsport.

Health Professionals Council

Society of Sports Therapists

British Association of Sport Rehabilitators and Trainers

Sports Massage Association

VTCT – specialist awarding body

ITEC – awarding organisiation for qualifications in beauty, complementary and sports therapy

Independent Professional Therapists International

Federation of Holistic Therapists

Physio Supplies Limited – physiotherapy, rehabilitation, and sports therapy equipment supplier

Physio-Med Services – physiotherapy and rehabilitation product suppler

Further reading

Brukner, P. and Khan, K. (2007). *Clinical Sports Medicine*. Sydney: McGraw Hill.

Cash, M. (1998). *Sport and Remedial Massage Therapy*. London: Ebury Press.

Grodzki, L. (2000). *Building Your Ideal Private Practice: A Guide for Therapists and Other Healing Professionals*. New York: WW Norton & Co.

Paine, T. (2007). *The Complete Guide to Sports Massage*. London: A&C Black.

Smith, A. and Stewart, B. (1999). *Sports Management: A Guide to Professional Practice*. Sydney: Allen & Unwin.

Ward, K. (2004). *Hands on Sports Therapy*. London: Thomson Learning.

Chapter 14

Study skills

Introduction

Being able to take in new information, retain it and tackle assessments efficiently and effectively can be facilitated with the proper use of study skills. These are strategies to enhance your learning, improve achievement and ultimately to help you succeed on your course.

This chapter introduces learning styles that will enable you to identify the right one for you. If you are aware of your preferred learning style you can choose the most effective way to study.

Attention and time should be devoted to developing your study skills, in order to facilitate your understanding and learning, and obtain the grades you deserve. Study skills covered in this chapter include the use of flash cards, listening skills, taking notes, reading skills and improving concentration.

This chapter covers skills to help you to prepare presentations, complete essays and revise for examinations.

Learning outcomes

After you have read this chapter you should be able to:

- identify and describe your learning style
- develop your study skills
- understand how to prepare for assessments.

Identify and describe your learning style

You will experience two types of learning throughout your course – pedagogy and andragogy. Pedagogy is teacher-led education; your lecturer will decide your learning content and best method of delivery. Andragogy is learner-focused education; this is where you are responsible for your own learning. This method is apparent in your self study and with your work experience module. To help you with your own learning you need to decide on your preferred learning style.

Table 14.1: Fleming (1995) suggests there are five learning styles

Learning style	Tools and activities	Mini activity
Visual learners (learn best through seeing)	• Use visual images – pictures, models, videos, flow charts, graphs and textbooks • Use different colours, highlight key information and underlining	• Select lecture notes and highlight key information in colour. • Can you display the information in a visual manner such as a flow chart?
Aural learner (learn best through listening)	• Attend lectures • Record lectures using a dictaphone and replay • Active participation in discussions and tutorials • Explain information to others • Describe visual information	• Ask permission from your lecturer to record a lecture using a dictaphone. • Now replay the lecture and fill in any gaps in your lecture notes.
Read/write (learn best through reading and writing)	• Read textbooks, journals and definitions • Write lecture notes up in full • Use headings, lists and definitions • Read lecture notes aloud	• Read several journals in relation to a lecture topic.
Kinaesthetic (learn best through experience)	• Focus on learning through moving, touching and doing • Visit medical school • Work experience placements • Shadowing other professionals	• Seek a placement in which you can shadow a sports therapist working.
Multimodel	• Learn via a combination of two or more learning styles	

Learning styles

One of the most widely used methods to identify different learning styles is the VARK model. It includes a series of questions and you choose the answer which best describes your preference. Your preferred learning style will be shown, and advice given about specific study strategies. By understanding your preferred learning style, you can use appropriate techniques to facilitate your learning.

To obtain a secure link to an online learning styles questionnaire, see the *Useful resources* list on page 186.

Develop your study skills

Good listening

To maximise your performance you need to be a good listener. Taught programmes are heavily reliant on the delivery of information and your ability to listen. Listening is a cognitive act that requires you to pay attention, think about the information delivered and mentally process it.

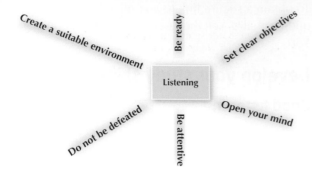

Figure 14.1: Key components to ensure you are a good listener. How can you achieve each of these?

- **Be ready** – read any notes before the lecture. Consider how much you already understand about the topic that is due to be delivered. Make a conscious effort to find the topic useful and interesting.

- **Clear objectives** – have a clear idea of what you expect from the lecture and the topic to be delivered. Ask questions if you are unsure of anything or if you think something has not been covered. Your lecturer may highlight that your question will be addressed in the next lecture.

- **Open your mind** – question what you are being taught but allow enough time for information to be covered. Your question may be answered as the lecture progresses. If it isn't, ask at a suitable interval, not in the middle of the lecture. Be receptive to new ideas and points of view.

- **Be attentive –** turn off your mobile phone so you are not tempted to surf the Internet or check for text messages. Focus, and maintain eye contact with your lecturer. Sit in a position where you can fully engage in the lecture and not be distracted by others.

- **Do not be defeated** and stop listening when you feel challenged or find a topic hard. This is the time to increase your focus and listen very carefully while opening your mind. If you are struggling to understand, say so – others are probably feeling the same.

- **Environment** – if the room is too hot, sit by an open window and if you know the room is cold, wear extra clothing. Be proactive and think how you can best cope with the environment to limit the distraction.

Make the most of lectures

Make the most of your lectures and you will gain a better understanding which could save you struggling later. Maximising your experience involves the following.

- **Preparation** – look on your university's virtual learning environment (VLE – your VLE may be referred to as a blackboard or moodle) and download the lecture notes and any required reading. Read them, reflect on the material and prepare questions. Take everything you need for making notes during the lecture.

- **Active participation** – make additional notes, listen attentively and ask questions to clarify where you are unsure. Try to understand the main message of the lecture and the links and ideas presented. Write key information quickly, particularly anything the lecturer has highlighted as important to your assessment or exam. If you know something requires further research, add a question mark to draw your attention to it after the lecture.

- **Closure after the lecture** – review your notes. Highlight information and rewrite, expanding on areas. Display information visually. Develop a system which works for you, and ensure you file in an organised way. Your notes will be a valuable resource when preparing for exams, assignments and further reading. Investing time now will save time during the assessment period and will develop your understanding of the subject. Complete any reading you are given to reinforce your understanding and make your notes more comprehensive.

Reading

Reading is an important part of your course, and can be time-consuming. You need to identify your purpose for reading materials and what you want to ascertain.

Study reading
- Use when reading more complex material
- Read more slowly than your normal reading pace
- May need to read more than once to understand the complexity.

Scan reading
- Use to quickly locate a specific piece of information
- Scan a paragraph or list to identify a specific piece of information.

Reading

Skim reading
- Use when you need to quickly obtain a general idea
- Identify the main ideas of each paragraph
- Read a large amount of material in a short time
- Lower level of comprehension.

Figure 14.2: The three reading styles: study reading, skim reading and scan reading. Identify where you can use each of these reading styles in your study.

Active reading helps to keep the mind focused on the task in hand. If you own the book, or have printed out a journal, highlight or underline important details as you read. It will help to keep you focused. You may also wish to annotate the reading to reinforce information and make points for revision. If you have borrowed a reading source and find particular parts useful, take a photocopy so you can mark it.

Critical thinking and approach

Being critical is a skill you need to develop. A critical approach means you do not accept ideas, information opinions and research at face value. You will question the approach, research methodology, assumptions and attitudes and discuss them within your work.

Thinking critically involves understanding the strengths and weaknesses of an argument, drawing conclusions, identifying any parallel arguments and judging how sound arguments are. When reviewing research think about the world view, the strategy taken, methodology and data as well as conclusions drawn. Within your work you will develop your critical thinking by making a claim; this will form the basis of your argument,

progressing to flaws in your argument and analysing strengths and weaknesses in relation to the evidence available. You will then question the evidence that is available.

Developing your critical thinking skills will improve your study skills. There are three main aspects to critical thinking – process, understand and analyse.

- **Process** – the taking in of information which you are reading, or which has been delivered to you.

- **Understand** – consolidate your understanding of the information by summarising key points or the evidence presented.

- **Analyse** – spend time thinking how all the components interrelate, and gain an in depth overview.

You need to understand the key words within your assessment brief. Throughout your course you will encounter words such as **evaluate**, **synthesise**, **apply**, **justify** and **compare**.

Flash cards

Flash cards can be very helpful, for example, when learning functional anatomy (for more information see *Chapter 1: Functional anatomy*). You can buy anatomical flash cards, or make your own with reference to any subject.

Key terms

Evaluate – this is an assessment of the information with regards to your topic, the evidence it is based on and its relation to other ideas

Synthesise – you should draw together information from a range of sources you have researched to support the assessment you are constructing. Logical connections should be made and presented in a logical format

Apply – this is the transference of information and knowledge you have gained to your topic, or application to practical aspects

Justify – the conclusion you have drawn or ideas you have formed will need to be justified. The information you have researched will allow you to support your work

Compare – you should address the similarities and differences presented in the information you have gathered

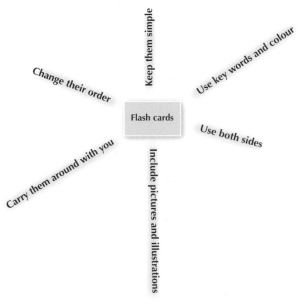

Figure 14.3: Key considerations when designing flash cards.

Flash cards are useful during group study. Take it in turns to randomly pick a card and then discuss subjects related to the flash card. This is a good method to practise for your viva voce (see page 183). You can also maximise your revision time when you have a spare 10 minutes, for example, when travelling on buses or trains.

Activity

Design a set of flash cards for a subject you are finding challenging.

Time management

Time management is essential if you are to produce good-quality work and achieve your grades. Your academic grades are a measure of your success, are rewarding and can provide you with the motivation to succeed. Poor time management often lets students down, resulting in poor grades.

A schedule reflecting the semester will help you to see the big picture. Your university will provide you with a course handbook or module handbook. This will tell you how many assessments you will have for the module, the types of assessment you will have (for example, presentation, essay, viva voce or examination) and the dates for submission. Develop a calendar for the semester and, for each module, list the type of assessment and the submission date. This will allow you to reflect on the semester ahead, what is expected of you and when you can expect a greater workload.

Planning a weekly schedule, reflecting on both academic and personal tasks, is invaluable in improving your time management. On a seven day diary, from getting up to going to bed, document your typical week including:

- work commitments
- sports training and matches
- timetabled lectures
- travel to and from work, university and training
- social activities
- late morning rising
- surfing the Internet, for example on Facebook and Twitter
- studying.

Have you allocated sufficient time to your studies? You may need to sacrifice some less urgent activities in order to plan your study time effectively. You may also need to increase the time scheduled which leads up to a busy assessment period.

To improve your time management consider:

- the time of day you study best
- studying difficult subjects first
- studying in an appropriate environment
- making use of a library when researching
- reviewing your schedule daily and weekly
- having clear objectives to achieve daily and weekly
- making a 'to do' list
- reflecting on your accomplishments.

If you are not achieving your 'to do' list, daily or weekly objectives, why not? Where is your time going? How can you manage your time more effectively?

Improve your concentration

Maintaining concentration while studying is a task in itself. There is always something to distract you – television, surfing the Internet, phone calls, making drinks, etc. Being able to concentrate and focus on the task in hand is essential. Consider the following to help improve your concentration:

- Remove all distractions and turn off your mobile phone – unplug the landline if necessary. Your environment should be quiet and at the right temperature. If you live in busy student accommodation it may be better to study in the library.
- Make a study plan. Confirm what you are trying to accomplish in the study session and how long it will take you. If you have a complex task, break it down into smaller tasks which are easier to accomplish.
- Study at the time of day which is best for you.
- Ensure you are in the right mind set. If you are tired and hungry you won't have the energy to concentrate.
- Work for 20 to 30 minutes interval periods and take regular breaks where you leave your study area.
- Ensure you have all the materials you require to study, including academic texts, journals and basic writing materials.

Motivation

Every student will find it difficult to motivate themselves at times. A lack of motivation will affect your concentration, focus and attitude. You may become negative and begin to feel the challenge is insurmountable. You will often find every excuse to avoid studying.

Motivation is the key to a positive attitude and believing you can achieve. Motivated students will find it easier to focus and improve their learning. Consider the following to improve your motivation.

- Use the 'concentration' list above to stay focused.
- Study with colleagues. Group study can be just as beneficial as individual study.
- Tick off aspects on your study plan when you accomplish them – this can be very rewarding.
- Focus on the long-term goal of achieving your foundation degree or Higher National.
- Remember you have actually paid for this course. Pin your receipt somewhere obvious to remind you of the cost.
- The sooner you start the sooner you will finish. If you spend time worrying about studying and avoiding the issue, you are losing valuable study time.

How to prepare for assessments

You will need to complete several assessments during your course. Read the assessment brief carefully and understand the task/s fully. If you are unsure, ask your tutor. Pay particular attention to the reading list on the assessment brief. Key readings will have been included to develop your understanding.

Preparing for a presentation

In sports therapy you must be able to communicate effectively with a range of people and explain and justify your decisions. At some point during your career you will be expected to present information. You need a good understanding of your presentation topic to be able to communicate effectively with your audience and answer any related questions.

Table 14.2: Top tips for an effective presentation

Preparation	Carry out research and understand your subject area thoroughly. Practise your presentation a number of times before your assessment. You could video yourself and reflect on your performance, or practise with colleagues and ask for feedback. Answer the task you have been given, and time yourself to ensure you stay within the time limit.
Presentation	Prepare your slides using a suitable IT package, for example PowerPoint® or www.Prezi.com. Ensure your material is presented with clarity, referenced and has visual aids. Do not overload your slides with lots of text which you are tempted to read word for word.
Your presentation	Dress appropriately. Present a positive attitude conveying enthusiasm and confidence.
Examples	Provide a range of examples to help explain aspects, ensuring they are related to the subject.
Additional aids	Use additional aids such as anatomical models, props or handouts to help support your explanation.
Audience	Connect with your audience by maintaining eye contact with them. Scan all participants in the audience.
Interesting	Make your presentation interesting by using visual aids. Ask questions to involve the audience (ensuring they are at an appropriate level). If you use video clips keep them short (20–30 seconds maximum) and clearly state their purpose or relevance.
Voice	Speak at an appropriate speed and vary the tone of your voice.

Exam

In order to prepare effectively for examinations allow adequate time. Implement good time management throughout the process, make a concerted effort and persevere through any difficulties.

Write down the exam date, time and location on your semester calendar and produce a revision schedule to meet the exam deadline.

Top tip

Remember KISS : **K**eep **I**t **S**imple and **S**traightforward. Start with the basics and progress to more complex information.

When revising, refer back to the list on page 181.

Maintain a routine before the exam, including regular meals to keep up your energy levels. If your exam is in the afternoon do not 'cram' in the morning – just refresh your memory with key points. Have a good night's sleep before a morning exam, and a final read through of revision notes. Ensure you have all your equipment and arrive in plenty of time for the start of the exam.

During the exam read the instructions carefully, and read *all* the questions first to identify those which are compulsory and those which are optional. Plan how much time you will allocate to each question, allowing a proportion of time to read through your answers. Clearly identify your answers within your answer book and start with the question you feel most confident with.

Use all your time – never leave an exam early. Ensure you have answered the correct number of questions and your answer matches the question number. Read through your answers and edit where necessary, but remember it's about the quality of your work, not the quantity. If you are running short of time, list the key information. Take care that your handwriting is legible – if the examiner cannot read your work they cannot mark it.

Writing an essay

An essay is structured by using coherent paragraphs which are connected in a logical way. An introduction is used to introduce the essay topic, with the main body developing an argument, linking point 1 to point 2, to point 3, etc. Always end your essay with a conclusion. This should conclude your argument and summarise the main points of the essay.

An essay takes time to develop. For a 2500 word essay allow a minimum of three weeks; for longer essays allow more time. This time is not just to write the essay, it is for planning, drafting and redrafting, as well as editing and refining your work, paying particular attention to your spelling, grammar and referencing. The essay writing process can be broken down.

1. **Understand the topic** – ensure you fully understand the essay topic and the requirements of your work. Identify the key words within the essay title and make sure you understand their full meaning. You need a full grasp of the topic in order to ensure that all the information you include is relevant. You may decide to formulate your argument to the topic in question, in order to provide direction for the planning process. You can always amend your argument as your knowledge develops. Highlight key information on the assessment brief you have been given.

2. **Thought shower** – this will allow you to put down all your ideas. Think laterally and document all information, even if something seems irrelevant (you may make a connection later on in your work). A thought shower will help you to focus on your plan and reading.

3. **Essay plan** – produce a plan for your essay. Think about the structure and which topics you are going to put where, and in what order.

4. **Reading** – read a wide range of sources related to your essay topic and plan – use books as well as academic journals. The Internet is a good source to develop thoughts and ideas and gain a quick understanding but should rarely be used as an academic reference. Academic references should form the basis of your research; these include books and journals.

5. **Amend essay plan** – on completion of your reading you will have a better understanding of the topic. Review your plan and make any amendments. Do you need to move or add a topic? Your plan should help you to write analytically. Consider the following points and amend your plan as necessary.

- Clearly identified main proposal, hypothesis or argument.

- Reasoned argument considering evidence, examples and research.

- Reasoned opposing argument – again considering evidence, examples and research.

- Justification of your perspective – address weaknesses and flaws in opposing arguments evidence, examples and research.

6. **Draft 1** – you need to write your essay based on your plan and the reading you have completed. If you feel there are gaps, or you don't have sufficient information, make a note and address these when you have completed the first draft.

7. **Additional information** – your first draft will have allowed you to ascertain weaker areas, and areas which require further understanding. Focus your additional reading on these areas.

8. **Draft 2** – amend your first draft to address any weak areas or gaps in your work.

9. **Break** – take a break from your work. Fresh eyes and thought will enhance the next stage.

10. **Final version** – review your work focusing on the flow and logical structure. You may need additional sentences or paragraphs to improve the links. Is there any irrelevant information? Focus on each sentence. Could you write the sentence with fewer words or with a clearer structure?

11. **Proofreading** – this is the final read through paying particular attention to details such as spelling, punctuation and referencing. A third party could always help with this stage of your essay. Referencing within the text as well as including a full reference list is often overlooked by many students. The section on referencing on page 184 includes details.

Viva voce examinations

Viva voce are included as an assessment strategy in most courses. With an essay you have access to many resources which you can collate, and time to reflect and amend your work. With a viva voce it is crucial you understand your subject area and are able to communicate information confidently and logically to your examiner. You will not pass by reciting information you have learned verbatim. Prepare thoroughly for your viva voce.

- Be logical. Start with the basics and progress to more complex information. For example, the practical may require you to palpate a bony prominence, and demonstrate ligament tests to the associated joint. Your viva should be logical, starting with the basics and identifying the ligaments, progressing to discuss their origin and insertion, progressing to describe the associated joint and its structures, and then to the surrounding musculature, identifying individual muscles actions, origins and insertions.

- Understand the requirements of your viva voce and draft possible questions you may be asked – you can then verbalise your answers.

- Use anatomical models to verbally explain information – this will allow you to ascertain your understanding.

- Revise and practise with other students.

Top tip

- Be prepared and wear your sports therapy uniform unless you are instructed to wear smart professional attire.

- Stay calm and pleasant and maintain an appropriate manner and attitude.

- Listen carefully to the question. Don't be afraid to ask the examiner to repeat it.

- If you don't know the answer, do not bluff – acknowledge that you don't know.

- Do not worry if parts of the viva voce were difficult. The examiner will ask a range of questions differing in complexity and difficulty in order to ascertain your knowledge and grade.

Referencing

In order to inform your assessment, your work needs to be based on academic sources. The material you read and research will form the substance of your work. Making reference to another author's work is known as citing and you must give a full detailed list of all sources used in a reference list at the end of your work. You must fully reference your work, if you do not you may be guilty of plagiarism.

Your university or college will have their own referencing guide which may differ slightly from the examples below. Pay particular attention to detail. This can be a time-consuming process so on completion of your assessment, allow time in your planning.

When you are making direct reference to an author's original idea, or a study they have conducted, reference as follows:

Paine (2000) states that...

Ylinen and Cash (1996) propose that...

If there are more than four authors for the publication you should cite them as follows:

Marra et al. (2002) state that...

When you are not directly making reference to an author, although you have used their concepts or ideas, you should reference as follows:

Sports massage has both physiological and psychological benefits (Paine, 2000).

If you have identified two sources which support this idea you should reference as follows:

Sports massage has both physiological and psychological benefits (Ylinen & Cash, 1996; Paine et al., 2002).

The references at the end of your essay should be in alphabetical order. To reference a book, follow this format:

Paine, T. (2000). *The Complete Guide to Sports Massage*. London: A&C Black.

To reference a journal, follow this format:

Sharma, P. and Maffulli, N. (2005). Tendon Injury and Tendinopathy: Healing and Repair. *Journal of Bone and Joint Surgery*, Vol. 87, 187–202.

Top tip

If you have two publications from the same author for the same year you should distinguish by placing an 'a', 'b' after each of the years. For example, Mackay (2010a) and Mackay (2010b).

Plagarism

Plagarism is copying someone else's work or passing their work off as your own, or taking ownership of their original ideas. If you quote material and do not put it into quotation marks, or fail to reference the source, this is classed as plagiarism. This is taken very seriously and may lead to disciplinary proceedings. Most universities and colleges will provide you with access to plagiarism detection software called Turnitin. Turnitin is a tool you can use to gain feedback on the potential of plagiarism within your work and improper citation. It can be used at any stage of your work, for example at first draft, second draft and your final version. Turnitin allows you to be proactive to avoid any plagiarism issues. You will find it on your college's or university's VLE. All work is submitted electronically.

Taking responsibility

There is only one person responsible for your learning and achievement on your course, and that's you. It's easy to blame others or make excuses but you need to take responsibility for your learning, be proactive and find constructive solutions. Some of the following might sound familiar:

- I can't do it, it's too difficult…

- It won't work… it's a waste of time… it's doing my head in…

- It's not my problem… it's not fair…

You might hear or say:

- They didn't explain it properly…

- They should help me more…

- It's their fault…

- They have to do something about it…

Take responsibility for a constructive outcome. Use phrases such as:

- I can do this…

- I don't fully understand the lecture therefore I am going to…

- I will take responsibility for…

- It is my fault I did not do as I was asked so next time I will…

- I have not completed the required reading so next time I will…

Be positive, be proactive and plan to achieve.

Universities have many support systems in place that you can use as much as you need to.

Time to reflect

1. Use an online questionnaire to identify your learning style. Describe the methods that will help you to learn more effectively. To obtain a secure link to an online learning styles questionnaire, see the Useful resources list on page 186.

2. Briefly describe two strategies which you could use to improve your listening skills.

3. Identify the three reading strategies and briefly describe why you would use each.

4. Choose two strategies which you could use to maximise the use of your lectures.

5. Discuss which topic you could design flash cards for and how this would enhance your learning.

6. Discuss two ways you could improve your concentration when studying.

7. Discuss two strategies you could use to improve your motivation.

8. Discuss three aspects to consider when preparing for a presentation.

9. Identity the 12 stages of writing an essay.

10. Discuss why it is important to take responsibility for your own learning.

Useful resources

To obtain a secure link to the websites below, see the Websites section on page ii or visit the companion website at www.pearsonfe.co.uk/foundationsinsport.

VARK learning styles questionnaire

Information about Disabled Students' Allowances (DSAs) from Directgov

Dyslexia at College – for dyslexic students at college or university

BRAINHE – resources for learning with specific learning difficulties

Epax – study skills online

Learn Higher – Centre for Excellence in Teaching and Learning

Essay writing skills from the Study and Learning Centre at RMIT University

Skills4Study from Palgrave Macmillan

Learning Space Skills Forum from the Open University

Further reading

du Boulay, D. (2009). *Study Skills for Dummies*. Chichester: John Wiley & Sons.

Cotterall, S. (2008). *The Study Skills Handbook*. Basingstoke: Palgrave Macmillan.

Greetham, B. (2008). *How to Write Better Essays*. Basingstoke: Palgrave Macmillan.

Cotterall, S. (2011). *Critical Thinking Skills*. Basingstoke: Palgrave Macmillan.

Fleming, N.D. (1995), I'm different; not dumb. Modes of presentation (VARK) in the tertiary classroom, in Zelmer, A. (Ed) *Research and Development in Higher Education, Proceedings of the Annual Conference of HERDSA*, HERDSA, Vol. 18, 308–313

Chapter 15

Work-based learning

Introduction

Work-based learning allows you to integrate theoretical knowledge with the practicalities of a workplace setting. Most universities will have their own student led clinic which is open to the public, enabling you to work supervised within an educational and commercial sports therapy setting. Support will be given to develop your clinic and pitch side skills to industry standards. This is important to prepare you for your industrial placement. *Chapter 16: Industrial placement* will support you through your industrial experience.

Within the clinic setting you will be responsible for completing a minimum of 40 hours of treatments. You will be required to draw upon your knowledge to identify and implement protocols such as subjective and objective consultation, analyse your findings to identify and implement treatment strategies, as well as recommending appropriate aftercare advice. During your pitch side experience you will be able to implement your first aid knowledge and skills.

This chapter will clarify employment opportunities, possible roles you may undertake in employment, as well as verbal and non-verbal communication skills. Personal skills will be addressed to further develop your knowledge and practice.

Learning outcomes

After you have read this chapter you should be able to:

- discuss employment opportunities for sports therapists
- explain the roles a sports therapist may undertake within the industry
- demonstrate knowledge of appropriate verbal and non-verbal communication skills
- discuss personal skills essential for employment.

Employment opportunities for sports therapists

Sports therapy has developed substantially over the past decade with new employment opportunities arising all the time. There is a variety of opportunities available and a high proportion of sports therapists work within the field on a self-employed basis. For several years you may work part-time and work unsociable hours. Being self-employed means you work for yourself and are responsible for all aspects of your business, including seeking job opportunities, tax returns, paying National Insurance and record keeping. You won't receive benefits such as sick pay and a private company pension. However, you do choose your own hours of work and the type of work you wish to undertake.

Many sports therapists undertake voluntary work while studying and upon qualifying, to ensure they have the relevant work experience to develop their personal profile and **curriculum vitae**. The disadvantage of voluntary work is that you will not be paid. However, reasonable expenses can usually be claimed. Volunteering is a good opportunity for you to network and gain valuable experience.

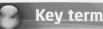

Key term

Curriculum vitae – document which provides an overview of your qualifications, employment and life

Roles a sports therapist may undertake

Your role will vary depending on your chosen employment. If you work within a sports club you will utilise your pitch side skills considerably more than in a clinic-based role. Should you seek employment with a low league sports team or become self-employed, you may be required to undertake a variety of roles including nutritional advice, sports psychology, advising on fitness and training programmes, as well as pre-season screening. If you work for a larger organisation or a professional team, you are more likely to work as part of a multi disciplinary team (MDT). Your role will be specific and you will be expected to liaise with different colleagues who might include the nutritionist, psychologist, fitness coach, strength and conditioning coach, physiotherapist and the medical team. Take time to ensure you clearly understand your role within your employment setting.

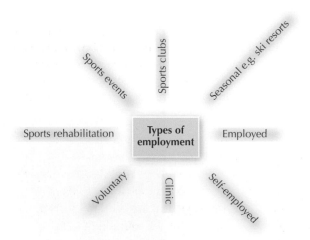

Figure 15.1: Types of employment – how would your role as a sports therapist differ between the employment opportunities?

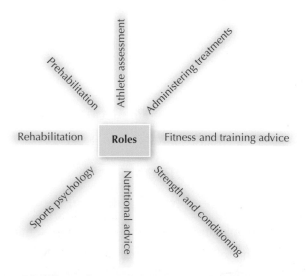

Figure 15.2: Examples of roles a sports therapist may undertake

Your foundation degree or Higher National will develop your portfolio of transferable skills. These are skills which can be applied to a range of jobs. Examples include communication, problem solving, leadership and time management.

> ● **Stop and think**
>
> Investigate your local area identifying all sports therapy jobs. Which roles do the jobs include?

Verbal and non-verbal communication skills

Good communication skills are essential if you are to develop successful relationships with clients, colleagues and employers. Good communication is important for you to convey your message to the recipient clearly and unambiguously. It is also essential that you receive information clearly. Any distortion to or from the sender will cause confusion and affect the treatment process or relations between those involved. Poor communication may result in loss of clients, job opportunities and lead to a poor reputation. There are two types of communication – verbal and non-verbal.

Verbal communication

Convey your message as clearly as possible to the recipient and avoid unnecessary jargon, for example complex medical terminology. Speak clearly, concisely and at an appropriate speed. Words should be chosen which convey your intent and deliver succinct meaning in a logical manner. It is essential you avoid creating resistance or a defensive mindset in your recipient. Avoid words which are accusatory, judgemental, blaming or critical.

Non-verbal communication

Research demonstrates that a high proportion of communication is non-verbal (this is more commonly known as body language). Body language includes eye contact, facial expressions, gestures, posture, voice, touch and space. Non-verbal communication is a powerful tool which you can use to secure employment, build rapport with clients, develop your client base and address challenging situations.

- **Eye contact** – to portray confidence ensure frequent eye contact. When first approaching the recipient make gentle eye contact, and develop the gaze. Intense eye contact is as detrimental as too little.

- **Voice** – think about the quality and projection of your voice, pace, expression and emphasis.

- **Posture** – move confidently, adopting a confident posture. This will make you feel more confident and make your client feel confident about you.

- **Facial expression** – your face is very expressive and communicates a wide range of emotions such as happiness, sadness, anger, fear and disgust. You should be aware of your emotional state and ensure you only show a positive, confident and pleasing expression.

- **Gestures** – many people talk with their hands, some more than others. Ensure that any hand gestures you make are not misinterpreted.

- **Touch** is used as a way to communicate. A clear distinction should be made between personal and professional communication. A firm handshake is a professional reassuring approach upon first meeting. A warm hug would be far too familiar and unprofessional within the work environment (although an appropriate way to greet a good friend).

- **Space** – the need for personal space differs from person to person. Invading a person's space can communicate signals for intimacy, aggression or dominance, all of which are inappropriate. Maintain your own personal space and respect the space of your client.

Effective and successful communication will depend on your ability to self-reflect, be emotionally self-aware and your ability to critique your own non-verbal communication skills in relation to the message you are sending out. Pay attention and be attentive to your client to fully understand the message they are conveying. A good way to hone your skills is to observe yourself in action through a digital recording (ensure you have the consent of your client). Watch your performance while identifying your strengths and any areas for improvement. Reflective learning will be addressed in *Chapter 16: Industrial placement*.

Personal skills required for employment

Chapters 1 to 13 focused upon the knowledge, understanding and practical requirements which you need to be a successful sports therapist. This section addresses those additional personal skills required for employment within the industry. Focus on implementing and developing these skills during your work-based learning so they are seamless during your industrial placement.

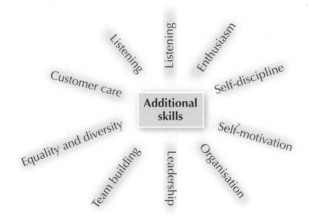

Figure 15.3: Additional personal skills required for employment

Listening

Listening is one of the most important skills a therapist can have. Your ability to listen to your clients will have a major impact on how effective you are as a therapist, as well as the quality of relationships you form. Listening enables you to learn, understand and obtain information.

Research suggests that you remember 25 to 50 per cent of the information presented to you. During a 30-minute consultation, you can surmise you will listen to between approximately 7.5 to 15 minutes only.

Stop and think

When you are listening during a consultation, how much information do you really hear?

By developing your listening skills, you can improve your productivity and negotiation skills, as well as avoid any misunderstanding and conflict.

Enthusiasm

Enthusiasm is paramount. It is the energy that you create to bring about a successful future. To have enthusiasm you need to have an interest in your subject and a knowledge and belief in yourself. Always be enthusiastic, but also realistic about what you and your clients can achieve. People don't gravitate towards boring people. Enthusiasm can act like a magnet, and people tend to be drawn to those who are enthusiastic because they are upbeat and positive. However, overenthusiastic people can be too intense, invade the recipient's space and repel others.

Self-discipline

Self-discipline is an important tool whether you are employed or self-employed. It is the ability, regardless of emotional state, to take action. Actions will vary from being punctual, professional practice and preparation to developing new behaviour and thought patterns. It is your ability to use your willpower to accomplish an objective, despite wishing you were doing something else. Self-discipline can be developed and trained.

Self-motivation

Self-motivation is your ability to motivate yourself. You will have a reason to accomplish an objective and find the strength to achieve without the need for persuasion or support from others. It is the ability to be able to motivate yourself to overcome setbacks, unfair criticism, overcome others' negative attitudes towards you and general resistance and barriers in life and at work.

Organisation

Organisation is the ability to plan and co-ordinate your personal and professional schedules. Many professionals can help, for example:

- a life coach can help organise life issues
- a secretary can help with time management
- a psychologist can help to manage the mind.

However, you will be required to take responsibility for all organisational matters. Having good organisation skills will help to improve aspects such as productivity, success, creativity, efficient working practices and cost-effectiveness.

Leadership

A leader is someone who guides and inspires, and sets a new direction and vision for others. This is important within the workplace, particularly if you are working as part of a multi disciplinary team. It is an essential component of your client relationship to lead you both to the intended goal. To be a good leader you need to make sure that everyone involved understands their role, and is included when goals are being set.

Team building

Team building is an essential skill for any manager or leader. Building a strong relationship between team members improves productivity and thus team success. To be able to do this you must understand each and every one of your team in terms of strengths, weaknesses and personalities. You must draw upon your leadership and motivational skills in order to develop the ability to work as a team.

Equality and diversity

Equality and diversity should be embraced and embedded. Equality gives every individual the opportunity to achieve their potential. This should be done free from any prejudice and discrimination to develop a fairer society. Diversity is about recognising individual or group differences, treating accordingly and valuing positively.

Customer care

Customer care is fundamental in any business. It involves ensuring that systems are in place to maximise client satisfaction, and that the team are trained to deal appropriately with customers. If you are self-employed this fundamentally lies with you. Excellent customer care is vital to your sales, for example client bookings, and thus links directly to profit. Profitability is dependent on customer service.

Stop and think

When have you received good customer care? Why was the care you received as a customer good? When have you received poor customer care and why was it poor? Would you return as a customer?

Time to reflect

1. Identify eight employed sports therapy job opportunities within your area.

2. Identify the roles you need to undertake as a self-employed sports therapist.

3. Identify the roles you would undertake working as part of a large multi disciplinary team.

4. Discuss why good communication skills are important.

5. Identify seven components of non-verbal communication. Discuss four components.

6. Briefly discuss eight personal skills a therapist needs to gain employment.

7. Discuss the additional skill of listening.

8. Define equality.

9. Reflect on your own practice and identify six strengths.

10. Reflect on your own practice. Identify four areas needing improvement and set yourself actions for improvement.

To obtain answers to these questions visit the companion website at www.pearsonfe.co.uk/foundationsinsport

Useful resources

To obtain a secure link to the websites below, see the Websites section on page ii or visit the companion website at www.pearsonfe.co.uk/foundationsinsport.

Business Link

Mind Tools – essential skills for an excellent career

Further reading

Brounstein, M. (2001). *Communicating Effectively for Dummies*. Chichester: John Wiley & Sons.

Cook, S. (2008). *Customer Care Excellence: How to create an effective customer focus*. London: Kogan Page.

Grodzki, L. (2000). *Building Your Ideal Private Practice: A Guide for Therapists and Other Healing Professionals*. New York: WW. Norton & Co.

Leland, K. and Bailey, K. (2006). *Customer Service for Dummies*. Chichester: John Wiley & Sons.

Paine, T. (2007). *The Complete Guide to Sports Massage*. London: A & C Black.

Smith, A. and Stewart, B. (1999). *Sports Management: A Guide to Professional Practice*. Oxford: Allen & Unwin.

Ward, K. (2004). *Hands on Sports Therapy*. London: Thomson Learning.

Chapter 16

Industrial placement

Introduction

Your industrial placement will allow you to put into practice your theoretical knowledge and techniques, along with the additional skills you explored in *Chapter 15: Work-based learning*. The organisation in which you complete your industrial placement will expect you to exhibit industry standards from the start, be proactive and have clear aims and objectives as regards your personal and professional development – and to be able to reflect on the latter.

Before you start any placement, your university or college will expect you to set targets, demonstrate the ability to engage in reflective practice throughout your placement using the Kolb learning cycle or Gibbs reflective cycle, and set new targets during your time in placement. It is particularly important that you develop your ability to reflect.

A key issue for you is to seek out opportunities to complete your work placement and to convince potential providers of the benefits they will gain by offering you an industrial placement.

This chapter will provide support when you are writing your letter of application and putting together your curriculum vitae. It will also help you to develop your knowledge and understanding of how to reflect upon your targets set and your experience of your placement.

Learning outcomes

After you have read this chapter you should be able to:

- write a letter of application
- write a curriculum vitae
- understand reflective practice
- describe Kolb's learning cycle
- describe Gibbs' reflective cycle.

Writing a letter of application

Potential workplace providers will receive many requests from students for placements so you need to make sure your letter is noticed. See Table 16.1 for some key points to remember.

Table 16.1: Dos and don'ts when requesting work placements

Do	Don't
• make your message clear	• use terms such as read now, urgent or help
• demonstrate a logical order representing your ideas and thoughts	• provide too much information – this will overload the reader
• proofread your letter for spelling and grammar	• use slang or abbreviations
• use the correct opening and closing phrase.	• be overfamiliar.

When you write a letter of application you should:

1. put your address at the top right-hand corner

2. place the address of the person you are writing to on the left hand side below your address

3. put the date below this on the right

4. always address your letter to somebody using their correct title, for example, Mr Cox or Ms Cox. Using first name terms to a person you don't know is too familiar and unprofessional. Using the title Mrs or Miss incorrectly can offend, therefore Ms is preferable. If you do not know the name of the person you are writing to you should address the letter Dear Sir or Madam

5. use your opening paragraph to convey the purpose of your letter; it is the most important element. Provide a clear, concise summary of your message, no longer than a couple of lines. Your letter should then go on to give information to support your message

6. structure your letter in a coherent manner. This is achieved by putting forward your ideas in structured sentences. These allow the reader to clearly understand each element of information being delivered. The sentences will be constructed in a logical order, therefore allowing the reader to formulate a complete picture of the message you are delivering. Make sure you use accurate spelling and correct grammar and sentence structure. Read your letter out loud to ensure that it reads correctly and flows well. Get another person to proofread your letter

7. use the last paragraph of your letter to state what you would like the person to do as a result of your letter and thank them

8. end your letter correctly. Use 'Yours sincerely' if you know the name of the person to whom you are writing, or 'Yours faithfully' if you do not.

Badgers Cottage
Lilliput lane
The Sidings
Little Harrowden
Bedfordshire
BE1 DG11

The Firs
10 Wintergreen Lane
Milford
Lancashire

18 June 2010

Dear Mr Cox or Dear Sir or Madam

Text of opening paragraph should provide a clear summary.

The main body of your letter should be well structured and your last paragraph should state what you would like the person to do.

Yours sincerely or Yours faithfully

Your signature

Your name typed

Figure 16.1: Template for a letter of application

Writing a curriculum vitae (CV)

A CV is known as a resumé, and is a logical overview of your working life. It is important to ensure your potential work placement provider notices you. It must be concise and accurate and needs to be thorough to highlight all relevant information. You should view your CV as your chance to sell yourself to your potential work placement provider. You are selling your skills, qualifications, experience and ultimately your ability to contribute to the organisation.

Many CV templates are available on the Internet for free but there is no perfect one. CV format will differ from person to person and situation to situation. The CV you construct for your work placement will differ from that of someone who has more years of experience and qualifications than you and who is applying for a job.

Consider how relevant information is when you are constructing your CV, and whether or not it will help you to sell yourself to the prospective organisation. What you must not do is draw attention to your weaknesses. For example, if you have a valid driving licence then this could be an advantage so include it on your CV. However, if you do not have a driving licence or have failed your test twice, do not include the information and draw attention to weaknesses.

Fundamental components to include in your CV are listed below.

- **Personal details**
  - Name.
  - Contact details – ensure these are personal details and not work details. Phone numbers included should be those which you are most accessible on. Email is a very accessible communication method.
  - NB Nationality is not required.

- **Education**
  - Include clearly the qualification and year of study (the institution is optional). Present the information starting with the most recent. For example:

September 2008 – June 2010, FdSc Sports Therapy, Distinction, University name

  - Include further education and school education. You may or may not wish to highlight GCSE grades.
  - If you have additional qualifications which are vocationally related, such as coaching, umpiring or first aid qualifications, you may wish to include a heading 'Vocational qualifications', particularly if you have a strong educational background. This will further sell your skills and abilities. If your education is weak and you have not entered into too much detail, you should include other qualifications here. This will enhance your education section and appear stronger to the prospective organisation.

- **Experience**
  - List all relevant experience you have gained. Include all employment and be prepared to be questioned on any gaps in your employment.
  - If you do not have an extensive employment history highlight experiences such as a gap year experience, part-time employment, voluntary work, charity work, summer camps, unpaid work, internships or association memberships. Provide a concise description of your experience for each.
  - If your employment history is extensive and you have additional experiences to offer you may wish to use the headings 'Employment history' and 'Experiences' to strengthen your CV.

Additional information and sections you may want to include in your CV are:

- **Personal details**
  - Marital status and family – this is optional
  - Date of birth – again, this is optional (age discrimination is illegal in the recruitment process under the Employment Equality (age) regulations 2006)

- **Personal statement**

  This should grab the reader's attention. It should detail your attributes and goals and be no longer than 50 words. If you have a strong CV you could combine this section with your letter of application.

- **Skills**

  The skills you detail should be specific to the position for which you are applying and demonstrate that you would be a positive addition to the organisation. Provide a summary of job-related and transferable skills.

  - **Job-related** – these skills are related to the position for which you are applying and should be directly related to your industrial placement. For a summary look at the title of the chapters within this book.

  - **Transferable skills** – all foundation degrees and Higher Nationals have a wide range of transferable skills embedded into the programmes. Transferable skills include teamwork, synthesis and analysing information, presentation, communication and problem solving.

- **Hobbies and interests**

  This section highlights you as a person. Your hobbies and interests can reflect your motivation, personality traits and personal skills. This section should still be related to the position applied for and sell you in a positive light. If it doesn't you should think about omitting it from your CV.

- **References**

  Do not provide any references on your CV. If the organisation wants this information they will ask you for it, or ask for it to be detailed on an application form. They should ask your permission to contact your referees either before an interview or upon appointment. You would not want your current employer to be approached for a reference when they do not know you have applied for another job, particularly if you are not appointed. For your industrial placement you may wish to put your supervisor's contact details here as an exception to the rule.

Reflective practice

Reflective practice is about developing purposeful learning. It involves you looking at your experiences in more depth in order to learn for next time. It will develop your personal and professional growth and develop your ability to link theory and practice.

For your industrial placement you will be required to set targets and reflect upon your progress in achieving your targets, and your experiences during your placement. Reflective practice is essential to help you learn from your experience, and to develop. This process should be continuous, both on a personal and professional level.

There are many academic theories to facilitate your reflective practice. The most popular used by universities and colleges within the industrial placement module are Kolb's learning cycle and Gibbs' reflective cycle.

The Kolb learning cycle

In 1984 David Kolb published his learning styles model known by various names including Kolb's experiential learning theory, Kolb's learning styles inventory and the Kolb cycle. Kolb suggests four stages to his model which can be entered at any stage, although they must be followed in sequence thereafter to ensure learning takes place. The four stages are:

1. **Concrete experience** – the 'doing' phase. This is your experience while completing your industrial placement.

1. **Reflective observation** – the reflective process of your industrial experience. You will self reflect throughout the placement by keeping a log. You may also obtain feedback from your supervisor, colleagues, peers, players and clients. These aspects can be drawn together to give an overall reflection of your industrial placement. Note that reflection on its own is not sufficient; you could complete this stage for the next 15, 20 or 30 years of your sports therapy career and not develop personally and professionally.

2. **Abstract conceptualisation** – this stage allows you to review and draw conclusions from your reflection. It is accompanied by you carrying out further research within the field of sports therapy and more input from your lecturers and other developmental activities. This will help you to plan what you would do differently next time.

3. **Active experimentation** – this is where you implement your changes within your industrial experience and therefore continue the cycle into the concrete experience stage. This cycle is continuous and ongoing throughout your industrial experience.

Gibbs' reflective cycle

Developed by Professor Graham Gibbs, the Gibbs' reflective cycle (1988) consists of six stages. It is one of the few models which takes into account emotion.

1. **Description** – describe exactly what happened during your work placement. You should keep a detailed log of each day. Depending on the nature of your placement you may have a timetable to follow, for example you may see clients on the hour every hour, or you may have training sessions timetabled; if this is the case you may decide to describe each session individually rather than a whole day at a time.

2. **Feelings** – for each of your descriptions, document what you were thinking and feeling at the time. You may comment on how confident you felt – did you feel that you could not answer a question because of lack of knowledge or did you feel you could not communicate effectively with a client?

3. **Evaluation** – for each experience you should list points (both good and bad). For example, it may be good you were gaining pitch side experience, but it wasn't very good when you witnessed an open fracture during play, because the sight of blood made you feel ill and you were unsure what to do.

4. **Analysis** – analyse what sense you can make out of the situation. What does it mean? Using the open fracture example, you could analyse that your knowledge of dealing with open fractures is poor and due to your lack of experience the shock and sight of the injury made you feel unwell.

5. **Conclusion** – conclude and document what else you could have done, or perhaps should have done, during that experience.

6. **Action plan** – if the situation arose again, what would you do differently, and how will you adapt your practice in the light of this new understanding? For the open fracture example, you could set actions to include gaining more supervised pitch side experience and attending a refresher first aid course.

The cycle is only momentarily complete – should the situation arise again you will have developed personally and professionally to deal with the situation and the new event will become a focus of the reflective cycle. Development is a continuous process.

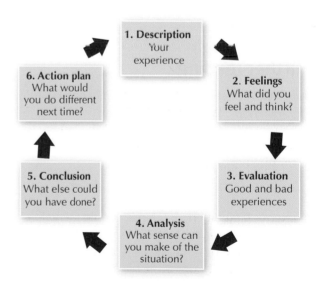

Figure 16.2: Gibbs' reflective cycle (adapted from Gibbs, 1988). Use the cycle to reflect on a recent sports match you competed in or a training session.

Time to reflect

1. Investigate five organisations where you could complete your industrial placement.

2. For each placement describe the skills you have to offer.

3. Write a letter of application for your chosen placement. Read the letter aloud and proofread, making any changes as necessary. Now ask a peer, friend or family member to proofread the letter, documenting any changes you need to make.

4. Discuss the headings which are fundamental to your CV.

5. Discuss the headings which are additional to your CV.

6. Construct a CV using an appropriate CV template from the Internet.

7. Summarise Kolb's learning cycle.

8. Summarise Gibbs' reflective cycle.

9. Choose which reflective cycle you are going to use to facilitate reflection during your industrial placement and provide a justification.

10. Use your chosen cycle to complete a reflection for a chosen activity.

To obtain answers to these questions visit the companion website at www.pearsonfe.co.uk/foundationsinsport

Useful resources

To obtain a secure link to the website below, see the Websites section on page ii or visit the companion website at www.pearsonfe.co.uk/foundationsinsport.

Business Link

Further reading

Boud, D., Cressey, P. and Docherty, P. (eds.) (2005). *Productive Reflection at Work: Learning for Changing Organizations*. London: Routledge.

Brounstein, M. (2001). *Communicating Effectively for Dummies*. Chichester: John Wiley & Sons.

Grodzki, L. (2000). *Building Your Ideal Private Practice: A Guide for Therapists and Other Healing Professionals*. New York: WW Norton & Co.

Ghaye, T., Cutherbert, S., Danai, K. and Dennis, D. (1996). *Learning Through Critical Reflective Practice. Self Supported Learning Experiences for Health Care Professionals*. Newcastle upon Tyne: Tyne Pentaxion Ltd.

Gibbs, G. (1988). *Learning By Doing: A Guide to Teaching and Learning Methods*. Oxford: Oxford Polytechnic.

Kolb, D. A. (1984). *Experiential Learning Experience as a Source of Learning and Development*. New Jersey: Prentice Hall.

Smith, A. and Stewart, B. (1999). *Sports Management: A Guide to Professional Practice*. Australia: Allen & Unwin.

Chapter 17

Case study: sports therapist

Context

Northampton Rugby Football Club is better known as the Saints. Their home ground is at Franklins Gardens. They compete in the premiership league and their rivals include Sale Sharks and London Irish.

The 1st XV coaches are Jim Mallinder (Director of Rugby), Paul Grayson and Dorian West. The performance team includes:

- Nick Johnston (performance director)
- Tom Bullough, Mark Finney and Chris Hart (conditioners)
- Dr David Cleal (team doctor)
- Matt Lee (lead physiotherapist)
- Sam Whiteson, Neil Fitzhenry and Caroline White (physiotherapists)
- Kiera Ruddy (masseuse).

Academy coaches include Dusty Hare (recruitment and development manager), Alan Dickens (academy manager) and Mark Hopley. For the full line up of who's who at the Saints, refer to the website listed in the *Useful resources* on page 203.

The stadium holds approximately 13,500, regularly selling out matches and averaging at 98 per cent capacity. The Saints have submitted an application to extend the stadium, increasing capacity to around 17,000. The stadium capacity needs to exceed 15,000 in order to meet the requirements of the organisers of the Heineken Cup to hold the quarter finals.

The sponsors of the Saints include Travis Perkins, Burrda, Church's English Shoes, Tetley's Bitter, Persimmon, Netgear, Hankook and Northampton Audi.

Meet Kiera

Kiera Ruddy, 22, began employment with the Saints in September 2009.

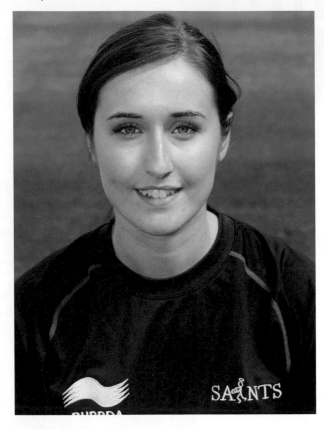

Her qualifications include:

- BSc Sports Therapy
- valid first aid certificate
- Level 1 APPI Pilates.

Continuous Professional Development:

- Pilates and the theraband course
- specific soft tissue mobilisations
- myofascial trigger points and muscular dysfunction.

Job description:

- accountable to the lead physiotherapist and performance director
- daily soft tissue treatment for players.

She is responsible for:

- pre-match soft tissue preparation
- post match and training recovery
- accompanying injured players to A&E in emergencies
- co-ordinating a bank of voluntary masseuses
- monitoring and ordering all tape and consumables
- providing Pilates sessions
- maintaining cleanliness of the physio room during and at the end of each day.

Background

Kiera has worked hard to attain her position as the sports massage therapist with the Northampton Rugby Football Club.

She began her studies in September 2006 at the University of Hertfordshire, reading for a BSc Sports Therapy degree. Work experience was a key component of the third year of the course. Kiera was a motivated and enthusiastic student, and was proactive in securing work experience with the Milton Keynes Dons Academy, shadowing the physiotherapist and actively participating at the Old Northamptonians RFC.

Experiences she gained at the MK Dons included injury assessment and diagnosis, injury rehabilitation, pitch side support and injury prevention. She learned about the importance of working within a multi disciplinary team and gained an insight into other professionals' roles. Kiera also learned that prevention of injury plays a major part in terms of prehabilitation. She continued to develop her portfolio of placements with Old Northamptonians RFC, gaining experience within a clinical setting and during pitch side duties. Work experience was invaluable and led to important personal and academic development. She also participated in a large number of clinical hours within the university sports therapy clinic, working under the supervision of qualified lecturers.

After graduating in June 2009 with a first class degree, Kiera made contact with the masseuse working at the Northampton Saints. The masseuse was looking for a sports therapy student to assist during the week and after home games. The commitment Kiera had already shown to her career proved vital and her hard work and passion for the job were rewarded. In September 2009 she was offered a part-time position on a consultancy basis as a sports massage therapist. This included attending games and developed into a full-time position.

Kiera feels strongly that sports therapy needs to be regulated and that those who have not trained to the benchmark standard, or who do not hold the appropriate insurance and membership of the regulatory body, should be barred from practice. She first purchased student membership of the Society of Sports Therapists in the first year of her degree and on graduating she upgraded to full membership for qualified practitioners. To meet with the insurance requirements, and ensure her emergency trauma care skills are competent, she has held a valid first aid certificate since her first year of training.

Kiera's responsibilities

Kiera reports directly to the head of performance and the lead physiotherapist. As a sports massage therapist, her responsibilities include:

- providing sports massage therapy:
  - to those players who require it
  - to injured players as part of their treatment programme
  - as a preventative strategy for players
- providing pre-game massage and massage during half time to the players who require it
- providing post game massage as part of the recovery session
- providing medical support to players who are injured during the game (e.g. ice, compression)
- being available for all home and away games
- providing 30-minute treatment sessions on the players' day off during the week
- instructing Pilates sessions as part of the core session to selected players twice a week
- providing additional Pilates sessions for players requiring stabilisation improvement
- managing all administration for the physiotherapy department.

Kiera liaises closely with the other medical professionals as part of a multi disciplinary team to enhance the players' well-being. If she feels that a player needs further treatment, she will tell them to book an appointment with the physiotherapist that day. She communicates this to the physiotherapist. If the physiotherapist is treating a player and believes they will benefit from additional sports massage treatments, the process is reciprocated. In addition the physiotherapist will communicate the area they require Kiera to work on and the expected outcome of the treatment.

The documentation of treatment notes is essential and required by law. Kiera is responsible for ensuring all players' records are comprehensive and kept up to date. The treatment notes are stored securely online in accordance with the Data Protection Act.

Kiera also ensures that the massage room adheres to health and safety and that cleanliness is maintained at all times.

A typical working day

Before training, treatments are conducted with players who have booked appointments. Any players with niggles, tightness or an injury are first assessed by the physiotherapist, and from there they are referred to Kiera for a loosen up before training if appropriate. While the players are in their first training session of the day, time is used efficiently, organising the physiotherapy room and completing any administration required. Any injured players are treated after they have completed their scheduled training.

Core training and flexibility sessions are conducted twice a week. During these, Kiera takes a small group of players through a challenging Pilate's session. Pilates was developed by Joseph Pilates early in the twentieth century; he believed in the use of the mind to control the muscles. Pilates is widely used both in sport and recreational training with the aim of developing strength, flexibility and body control.

The team holds a weekly discussion covering points such as which members of the team have played a high volume of games during the season (in particular forwards due to the nature of their game). Special emphasis is placed on particular players who need additional treatments. Lunchtimes are devoted to these players and those who have booked for maintenance sessions and flush outs before the next training session.

After lunch the players go into their second training session of the day and Kiera's schedule follows the same format as the first training session. At the end of the day, time is devoted to those players who may benefit from additional soft tissue manipulation. No day is ever the same, as all the players are different and require individual treatment. A positive team atmosphere is always developed.

At times, Kiera has to work unsocial hours including weekends and may sometimes work for several weeks without having a full day off, particularly pre-season. However, she loves her job, and enjoys supporting players in their recovery back to match play, maintaining their form during the season and eradicating those niggles and patches of tightness that players can experience.

Working in sport can be hard and you have to be prepared to put the hours in. You never stop learning. Within the next five years Kiera would like to study for an MSc in sports rehabilitation, and have completed the APPI (Australian physiotherapy and Pilates institute) Pilates and reformer training.

Injury scenario

A player has presented to Kiera with a pain in the buttock. During the past week there have been minor episodes of tingling in the gluteal region and pain is also prolonged when sitting for long periods. Kiera completes an assessment including active, passive and resisted movements in relation to the hip and vertebrae. There is a noticeable decrease in lateral rotation of the hip. Kiera summises piriformis syndrome. When piriformis shortens, lateral rotation is reduced and the sciatic nerve can be irritated. Piriformis release is a common treatment performed. The action of piriformis is to laterally rotate the extended thigh and abduct the flexed thigh. When running piriformis helps to keep the player upright as body weight shifts to the opposite side of the foot being lifted, and transmits force to propel them forward. Treatment performed is a piriformis release requiring the use of soft tissue mobilisation to elongate the fibres of the piriformis and thus increase range of movement. Muscle energy technique will be performed focusing on increasing lateral rotation. To complement the treatment over the next few days gluteal and hamstring stretches are prescribed as well as sitting on a tennis ball.

Describe how you would approach the treatment of the signs and symptoms.

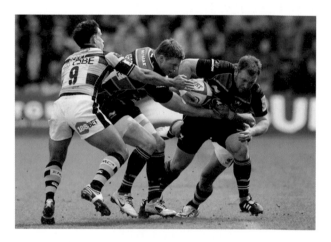

Figure 17.1: Kiera works hard to ensure that the Saints' team players are match fit

Time to reflect

1. Discuss the benchmark standard for a sports therapist.

2. Consider your personal strengths with regard to your ability to participate in reflective practice.

3. Consider your weaknesses with regard to your ability to participate in reflective practice.

4. Outline work placements which would be of benefit to you.

5. State five other teams that competed in the rugby premiership league season 2010–2011.

6. How does Kiera liaise with the physiotherapist?

7. What is the importance of the medical team meeting at the beginning of each week?

8. Investigate three organisations in your local area where you could complete a first aid at work qualification.

9. Investigate continuous professional development courses you may wish to undertake in the next couple of years.

10. Use the Internet to investigate Pilates and associated courses.

Useful resources

To obtain a secure link to the websites below, see the Websites section on page ii or visit the companion website at www.pearsonfe.co.uk/foundationsinsport.

Northampton Saints

Learning Space Skills Forum from the Open University

Skills4Study from Palgrave Macmillan

Australian Physiotherapy and Pilates Institute

Further reading

Boud, D., Keogh, R. and Walker, D. (1985). *Reflection: Turning Experience into Learning*. New York: Kogan Page.

Brounstein, M. (2001). *Communicating Effectively for Dummies*. Chichester: John Wiley & Sons.

Brukner, P. and Khan, K. (2007). Clinical Sports Medicine. London: McGraw Hill.

Ghaye, T., Cutherbert, S., Danai, K. and Dennis, D. (1996). *Learning Through Critical Reflective Practice. Self Supported Learning Experiences for Health Care Professionals*. Newcastle upon Tyne: Tyne Pentaxion Ltd.

Gibbs, G. (1988). *Learning by Doing: A Guide to Teaching and Learning Methods*. Oxford: Oxford Polytechnic.

Kolb, D. A. (1984). *Experiential Learning Experience as a Source of Learning and Development*. New Jersey: Prentice Hall.

Paine, T. (2007). *The Complete Guide to Sports Massage*. London:A & C Black.

Standring, S. (2008). *Gray's Anatomy: The Anatomical Basis of Clinical Practice, Expert Consult* (online and print). Edinburgh: Churchill Livingstone.

Ward, K. (2004). *Hands on Sports Therapy*. London: Thomson Learning.

Glossary

Absolute VO$_2$ max – maximal oxygen consumption expressed as l.min^{-1}

Adenosine tri-phosphate (ATP) – a high energy phosphate compound that is the body's only direct source of energy

Adherence – continuing to be physically active

Adhesions – bands of fibrous tissue formed between muscle fibres

Aetiology – the causes or mechanism of injury

Aftercare – includes any instruction given to a client to complete after the treatment (ideally in a written format)

Age predicted maximum heart rate – theoretical maximum heart rate calculated by 220 minus age

Agonist – the muscle producing the action (movement)

Amenorrhea – absence of the menstrual cycle without being pregnant

Anaerobic power – the ability to produce and maintain power output

Analgesic – a method of providing pain relief

Ankylosing spondylitis – an inflammatory arthritis affecting mainly the joints in the spine, sacroilium in the pelvis. However, other joints of the body may also be affected as well as tissues including the heart, eyes, lungs and kidneys.

Anorexia nervosa – an eating disorder associated with starvation of the body and excessive exercise

Antagonist – the muscle opposing the action (movement)

Anterior drawer test – a test performed with the knee in 90° flexion and the client's foot kept stable. The tibia is drawn forward and the joint is assessed for degree of movement and quality of end point

Anteriorly – towards the front

Aponeurosis – a flat, broad tendon

Appendicular skeleton – all the parts that are joined to the head and trunk (axial)

Apply – this is the transference of information and knowledge you have gained to your topic, or application to practical aspects

Articular cartilage – (also known as hyaline cartilage) is smooth and covers the surface of bones

Articulation – the contact of two or more bones at a specific location

Axial skeleton – the head and trunk of the body

Basal metabolic rate (BMR) – the amount of energy required to keep the body functioning at total rest

Bilateral – on both sides of the body, e.g. left and right leg

Bilateral comparison – the process of checking signs, symptoms and function on both the affected and non-affected side

Biomechanics – the study of forces and their effects on living systems

Bone mineral density (BMD) – the density of bones determined by mineral content

BORG scale – a scale of perceived exertion ranging from 6–20

Bradycardia – a resting heart rate below 60 beats per minute

Bulimia nervosa – an eating disorder associated with bingeing on food/drink and then purging through not eating, excessive exercise or laxative use

Cadence – the speed it takes to go through a full gait cycle

Chronic disease – diseases that an individual suffers with for months and years – they are long-lasting and recurrent

Closed kinetic chain – a movement chain in which the end of the chain is closed, i.e. in contact with the ground. Movement of one joint will produce movement of the other joints in the chain

Code of ethics – a set of professional behaviours or a set of formal rules and regulations often linked to a professional body

Cognitive appraisal – the way that we think about potentially stressful situations. This is linked to personality characteristics that influence the rehabilitation process and situational factors (sport, social and environmental factors that can influence injury rehabilitation)

Compare – you should address the similarities and differences presented in the information you have gathered

Concentric – muscle contraction generates force which causes muscle shortening

Contraindication – a condition or factor that speaks against a certain measure, medication or treatment

Costal cartilage – hyaline cartilage which connects the sternum to the ribs

Deformation – a change in a tissue's shape when subjected to a load (deformation to failure means the amount of deformation of a tissue when it reaches failure)

Delayed Onset of Muscle Soreness (DOMS) – pain and stiffness felt in muscles several hours to days after unaccustomed and/or strenuous exercise. Delayed onset muscle soreness begins 8–24 hours after exercise and peaks 24–72 hours after exercise (Marcora and Bosio, 2007)

Diaphysis – main shaft of the bone

Disability threshold – a threshold that determines an individual's autonomy and independence

Disaccharide – two monosaccharide molecules joined together. For example, sucrose is glucose and fructose bonded together

Distal – further away from the centre of the body

Diurnal variations – fluctuations which occur each day

Dorsiflex – move the top of the foot towards the body, showing the sole of the foot

Double support phase – the period of the gait cycle where support is being transferred from one foot to the other

Dypsnea – difficulty in breathing or shortness of breath

Eccentric – the muscle lengthens due to the opposing force being greater than the force generated by the muscle

Endomysium – connective tissue encasing individual muscle fibres

Enzymes – a type of protein with specific catalytic roles in metabolic reactions

Epimysium – connective tissue which encases all the fascicles surrounding the whole muscle

Evaluate – this is an assessment of the information with regards to your topic, the evidence it is based on and its relation to other ideas

Evert – move the sole of the foot away from the midline of the body

External imagery – imagining yourself doing something as though you are watching it on a film so that you can develop an awareness of how the activity looks

Fascia – fibrous tissue binding together or separating muscles

Fascicular arrangement – the arrangement of fascicles, which ultimately affects power output and range of movement

Fatigue – general sensations of tiredness and an accompanying reduction in mental and physical performance

Fibroblast – a cell in connective tissue

Fibrocartilage – this cartilage is very rich in type 1 collagen and is strong and durable. It can be found, for example, in the menisci of the knee and intevertebral disc

Fixator – provide stabilisation at the proximal end of the limb

Flight phase – the phase of the running gait where neither foot is in contact with the ground

Force – mechanical action or effort applied to a body that produces movement

Force transmission – impact forces transmitted through the body

Forced expiratory ratio – the ratio of FEV_1 to FVC

Forced expiratory volume – the percentage of vital capacity that can be expired in one second

Forced vital capacity – the amount of air that can be forcibly expired following a maximal inspiration

Frictions – small concentrated movements that can be applied in a circular or transverse motion, often used to help reduce scar tissue formation

Gait cycle – the time from heel strike of one foot to the next heel strike of the same foot

Glucose – a sugar that is the main form of carbohydrate used for fuel

Glycaemic index (GI) – the rate of digestion and absorption of carbohydrate, or how quickly carbohydrate eaten raises blood glucose levels

Glycogen – stored carbohydrate in the liver and muscles

Goniometry – the measuring of angles created by the bones of the body at the joints

Golgi tendon organ – located in the tendons that attach muscle to bone. The Golgi tendon organ provides information about muscle tension which is the semi-contracted state of a muscle over an extended period of time

Goniometry – the measuring of angles created by the bones of the body at the joints

Goniomoter – a device used to measure different joint angles

Ground reaction force – the equal and opposing force that is exerted by the ground on a body

Habitual physical activity – physical activity that is incorporated into everyday living

Haemoglobin – an iron containing pigments that binds oxygen to red blood cells

Hallux valgus – bunions

Hazard – a situation or object that could cause an accident or injury. For example, water on the floor is a hazard as it could cause someone to slip and fall

Health – the general condition of the body or mind, especially in terms of the presence or absence of illnesses, injuries or impairments

Homeostasis – the maintenance of a constant internal environment within the body

Hydrotherapy exercises – these are completed in water or a pool. They can be used in all the stages of injury and can add variety to the recovery programme

Hyperextension – extending a joint beyond its normal range of movement (it is associated with injury)

Hypertension – a chronic medical condition in which the systemic arterial blood pressure is elevated to a pressure of 140/90 mmHg or above

Hypertrophy – growth in size

Hypokinetic disease – chronic diseases associated with low levels of activity

Hyponatremia – a state of low plasma sodium concentration in the blood

Hypotension – low blood pressure 90/50 mmHg or below

Hypoxia – reduced pressure of inspired oxygen, thus reducing the amount of oxygen being sent to the tissues

Inertia – the resistance to changes in motion

Informed consent – informing your client by fully explaining the treatments to be administered

Injury aetiology – the study of how injury is caused or originates

Insertion – the attachment of a muscle usually via a tendon to bone. The insertion on the bone is moveable as a result of muscle contraction

Internal imagery – imagining yourself doing something and concentrating on how the activity feels

Intervertebral disc – a fibrocartilage disc which lies between each adjacent vertebrae of the spine

Invert – move the sole of the foot towards the midline of the body

Isometric – force is generated by the muscle contracting without changing length (i.e. without movement or when it is static)

Justify – the conclusion you have drawn or ideas you have formed will need to be justified. The information you have researched will allow you to support your work

Kilocalorie (kcal) – the amount of energy required to heat 1 litre of water by 1°C

Kinaesthetic awareness – a sensory skill that your body uses to know where it is in open space

Kinematics – the description of movements without reference to the forces involved

Kinetics – the assessment of movement with respect to the forces involved

Korotkoff sounds – the sounds that sports therapists listen for when measuring blood pressure using a mercury sphygmomanometer and stethoscope

Lachman's test – a test performed with the knee in 15° flexion where the examiner draws the tibia forward, assessing the joint for laxity

Lactate – a salt formed from lactic acid

Lactate threshold – the intensity of exercise where there is sustained increase in blood lactate above baseline values

Ligament – a band of tough fibrous tissue connecting bone to bone

Load – an external force

Lock – a lock is the firm pressure applied to an area of soft tissue to stop or limit movement

Lordosis – exaggerated curvature of the lumbar spine

Lymph – a fluid that carries water, electrolytes and proteins from the tissues

Lymph flow – the rate of supply and removal of lymph fluid

Lymphatic system – a network of vessels that carries lymph

Manual handling – when the body moves, usually lifting items, but it also includes pulling, twisting, pushing or climbing

Mass – the quantity of matter in a body

Mesomorph – a body type that is characterised by heavy, toned muscle content. The shoulders are broad, the thorax is large, the waist is quite slender and the abdominal muscles are defined

Mitochondria – an organelle found in cells and the site of aerobic energy production

Monosaccharide – a single sugar molecule. For example, glucose, fructose, galactose

Motor units – a motor nerve and all the muscle fibres it stimulates

Multi-factorial – caused by many factors

Negative self-talk – self-critical statements that can distract attention, reduce confidence and self-efficacy levels and make it harder to achieve goals

Neuromuscular junction – the site where a motor nerve communicates with a muscle fibre

Neutral vertebrae – the proper alignment of the body between postural extremes. In its natural alignment, the spine is not straight – it has natural curves in the thoracic (upper) and lumbar (lower) regions

Newton – force required to move a mass of 1 kg at a rate of $1 m.s^{-2}$

Occipital condyles – kidney-shaped with convex surfaces. There are two occipital condyles located either side of the foramen magnum. They articulate with the atlas bone

Omega-3 fats – polyunsaturated fats that particularly come from oily fish and seed sources and have a positive effect on health

Open kinetic chain – a movement in which one end of the chain is open, e.g. seated knee extension

Origin – the attachment site of a muscle to bone (in a few exceptions muscle). The origin is a fixed location

Orthotics – corrective insoles that can either be purchased over the counter or made by prescription, used to correct gait problems

Osteoporosis – accelerated deterioration of the weight bearing joints associated with ageing

Outcome goal – a goal that focuses on the outcome of an event

Outcome measures – using subjective and objective measures post treatment to evaluate and measure improvements

Overtraining – when the volume and intensity of training exceeds the body's ability to recover

Palpation – physical assessment of tissues using precise touching and feeling

Pathophysiology – the study of the changes of normal mechanical, physical, and bio-chemical functions

Performance goal – a goal that focuses on achieving performance objectives independent of other athletes

Perimysium – connective tissue encasing fascicles

Periodisation – the purposeful variation of a training programme over time, so an athlete achieves peak performance prior to an event or competition

Pes cavus – having a high foot arch

Pes planus –being flat footed with no noticable arch

Phosphocreatine (PCr) – an energy-rich compound that plays a role in providing energy by maintaining ATP levels

Placebo effect – a treatment which has no objective physiological benefit but which produces a subjective perception of a therapeutic effect

Plantarflex – point the toes away, pushing the sole of the foot away

Plyometric – a form of power training that involves eccentric actions followed by rapid concentric actions

Polysaccharide – a large chain of monosaccharides. For example, glycogen is a huge chain of glucose molecules

Positive self-talk – positive statements used to arouse and direct attention or to motivate people towards achieving goals

Prehabilitation – engaging in training and conditioning to deliberately reduce the chance of injury

Process goal – a goal that focuses on the actions that an individual must undertake to perform well

Progress – an injury getting better

Pronation – eversion, dorsiflexion and abduction of the ankle joint

Prone – laying face down

Proprioception – the body's awareness of its position in relation to other areas of the body and whether there is movement with required effort; also the body's ability to sense movements within joints and joint positions; also the body's ability to sense its positioning in open space and to determine the body's balance and stability

Proximal – towards the centre of the body

Quadriceps angle (Q-angle) – the angle between the line of the quadriceps muscle pull and the line of insertion of the patellar tendon

Regress – an injury getting worse

Relative VO$_2$ max – maximal oxygen consumption expressed relative to the client's body weight in kg and measured in $ml.kg.min^{-1}$

Respiratory exchange ratio (RER) – the ratio relating to volume of carbon dioxide expired to volume of oxygen consumed during activity

Risk – a risk is the likelihood that an accident might occur. For example, how likely is it that someone might slip on the water that has been spilled on the floor?

Sarcolemma – cell membrane of the muscle fibre

Sarcopenia – the process of lean tissue loss as we age

Sedentary – a state of being physically inactive

Self efficacy – the belief that an individual has in their own abilities to reach a specific goal or perform to a certain level

Serotonin – a hormone that causes changes in mood

Shear force – a force that often produces horizontal sliding of one layer of tissue over another

Shear stress – an internal resistance developed to a shear force

Soft tissues – a general term to describe tissues of the muscles, ligaments, and tendons

Stance phase – the phase of the gait cycle that begins with the strike of the heel on the ground (contact phase) and ends with the lift of the toe at the beginning of the swing phase of gait

Stressor – something that causes you stress, for example an injury

Stretch shortening cycle (SSC) – defined as an active stretch (eccentric contraction) of a muscle followed by an immediate shortening (concentric contraction) of that same muscle and determined by elastic potential of muscles and nervous innervation

Stroke volume – the amount of blood ejected from the heart in one beat

Supercompensation – positive adaptation made by the body following a period of training and recovery

Supinated – when the forearm is supinated the palm of the hand is facing forward when in the anatomical position

Supination – inversion, plantar flexion and adduction of the foot

Supine – laying down facing up

Sutural bone – extra piece of bone which appears in the suture in the cranium

Swing phase – the phase of the gait cycle where the foot is off the ground

Synergist – synergist muscles assist the agonist muscles and provide stabilisation to prevent any unwanted movement

Synovial fluid – fluid within synovial joints that lubricates the joint

Synthesise – you should draw together information from a range of sources you have researched to support the assessment you are constructing. Logical connections should be made and presented in a logical format

Tachycardia – a resting heart rate greater than 100 beats per minute

Tendon – a band of inelastic tissue connecting a muscle to bone

The Electricity at Work Regulations 1989 – also commonly known as portable appliance testing (PAT)

Thermic effect of activity – the effect of activity on metabolic rate

Thermic effect of food – the effect of food on metabolic rate

Thermogenesis – the process of heat production

Thrombosis – the formation of a blood clot inside a blood vessel, obstructing the flow of blood through the circulatory system

Torque – the turning effect or twisting motion created by a force about an axis

Transferable skills – general skills that can be used in any type of job

Transmitter fluid – a fluid that allows a nerve impulse to be carried across a neuromuscular junction to enable a muscle contraction

Valgus – the position in which a body segment is bowed laterally

Varus – the position in which a body segment is bowed medially

Vasodilation – an increase in the diameter of blood vessels that results in an increased blood flow

Venous return – the flow of blood back to the heart

VO_2 max – the maximum amount of oxygen that can be taken in and utilised by the body's working tissues in one minute; while breathing at sea level. VO_2 max is expressed as either absolute values in l/min or relative values in ml/kg/min

Index